# PATIENT'S AUTONOMY, PRIVACY AND INFORMED CONSENT

# Biomedical and Health Research

## Volume 40

*Earlier published in this series*

Vol. 8. M. Hallen and A. Klepsch (Eds.), Human Genome Analysis Programme

Vol. 9. A.-E. Baert, S.S. Baig, C. Bardoux, G.N. Fracchia, M. Hallen, O. Le Dour, M.C. Razquin, V. Thévenin, A. Vanvossel and M. Vidal (Eds.), European Union Biomedical and Health Research

Vol. 10. F.F. Cruz-Sánchez, R. Ravid and M.L. Cuzner (Eds.), Neuropathological Diagnostic Criteria for Brain Banking

Vol. 11. S.S. Baig (Ed.), Cancer Research at the European Level

Vol. 12. M. Maio (Ed.), Immunology of Human Melanoma

Vol. 13. V.K. Hopsu-Havu, M. Järvinen and H. Kirschke (Eds.), Proteolysis in Cell Functions

Vol. 14. G. ter Heege (Ed.), EURO-QUAL

Vol. 15. N. Katunuma, H. Kido, H. Fritz and J. Travis (Eds.), Medical Aspects of Proteases and Protease Inhibitors

Vol. 16. P.I. Haris and D. Chapman (Eds.), New Biomedical Materials

Vol. 17. J.J.F. Schroots, R. Fernandez-Ballesteros and G. Rudinger (Eds.), Aging in Europe

Vol. 18. R. Leidl (Ed.), Health Care and its Financing in the Single European Market

Vol. 19. P. Jenner and R. Demirdamar (Eds.), Dopamine Receptor Subtypes

Vol. 20. P.I. Haris and D. Chapman (Eds.), Biomembrane Structures

Vol. 21. N. Yoganandan, F.A. Pintar, S.J. Larson and A. Sances Jr. (Eds.), Frontiers in Head and Neck Trauma

Vol. 22. J. Matsoukas and T. Mavromoustakos (Eds.), Bioactive Peptides in Drug Discovery and Design: Medical Aspects

Vol. 23. M. Hallen (Ed.), Human Genome Analysis

Vol. 24. S.S. Baig (Ed.), Cancer Research Supported under BIOMED 1

Vol. 25. N.J. Gooderham (Ed.), Drug Metabolism: Towards the Next Millennium

Vol. 26. P. Jenner (Ed.), A Molecular Approach to Parkinson's Disease

Vol. 27. P.A. Frey and D.B. Northrop (Eds.), Enzymatic Mechanisms

Vol. 28. A.M.N. Gardner and R. Fox (Eds.), The Venous System in Health and Disease

Vol. 29. G. Pawelec (Ed.), EUCAMBIS: Immunology and Ageing in Europe

Vol. 30. J.-F. Stoltz, M. Singh and P. Riha, Hemorheology in Practice

Vol. 31. B.J. Njio, A. Stenvik, R.S. Ireland and B. Prahl-Andersen (Eds.), EURO-QUAL

Vol. 32. In production

Vol. 33. H.H. Goebel, S.E. Mole and B.D. Lake (Eds.), The Neuronal Ceroid Lipofuscinoses (Batten Disease)

Vol. 34. In production

Vol. 35. M. Schlaud (Ed.), Comparison and Harmonisation of Denominator Data for Primary Health Care Research in Countries of the European Community

Vol. 36. F.F. Parl, Estrogens, Estrogen Receptor and Breast Cancer

Vol. 37. J.M. Ntambi (Ed.), Adipocyte Biology and Hormone Signaling

Vol. 38. In production

Vol. 39. J.-Matthias Graf von der Schulenburg (Ed.), The Influence of Economic Evaluation Studies on Health Care Decision-Making

ISSN: 0929-6743

# Patient's Autonomy, Privacy and Informed Consent

H. Leino-Kilpi

M. Välimäki

M. Arndt

T. Dassen

M. Gasull

C. Lemonidou

P.A. Scott

G. Bansemir

E. Cabrera

H. Papaevangelou

J. Mc Parland

*IOS*
Press

Ohmsha

Amsterdam • Berlin • Oxford • Tokyo • Washington, DC

ISBN 1 58603 039 6 (IOS Press)
ISBN 4 274 90343 5 C3047 (Ohmsha)
Library of Congress Catalog Card Number: 00-100036


*Publisher*
IOS Press
Van Diemenstraat 94
1013 CN  Amsterdam
The Netherlands
fax: +31 20 620 3419
e-mail: order@iospress.nl


*Distributor in the UK and Ireland*
IOS Press/Lavis Marketing
73 Lime Walk
Headington
Oxford OX3 7AD
England
fax: +44 1865 75 0079

*Distributor in the USA and Canada*
IOS Press, Inc.
5795-G Burke Centre Parkway
Burke, VA 22015
USA
fax: +1 703 323 3668
e-mail: iosbooks@iospress.com


*Distributor in Germany*
IOS Press
Spandauer Strasse 2
D-10178 Berlin
Germany
fax: +49 30 242 3113

*Distributor in Japan*
Ohmsha, Ltd.
3-1 Kanda Nishiki-cho
Chiyoda-ku, Tokyo 101
Japan
fax: +81 3 3233 2426

# Authors

H. Leino-Kilpi, PhD, RN, Professor (University of Turku, Finland)

M. Välimäki, PhD, RN, Researcher (University of Turku, Finland)

M. Arndt, PhD, RN, Dipl. Rel. Päd., Dip. Phil., Consultant (Biomed project)

T. Dassen, PhD, RN, Professor (Humboldt Universität, Germany)

M. Gasull, RN (Escola Universitaria d'Infermeria, Hospital de la Santa Creu i Sant Pau, Spain)

C. Lemonidou, PhD, RN, Professor (National and Kapodistrian University of Athens, Greece)

P.A. Scott, PhD, RN, Senior Lecturer (University of Stirling, Scotland, UK)

G. Bansemir, PhD (Humboldt Universität, Germany)

E. Cabrera, RN (Escola Universitaria d'Infermeria, Hospital de la Santa Creu i Sant Pau, Spain)

H. Papaevangelou, Lawyer (Greece)

J. Mc Parland, RN, Doctoral Student (University of Stirling, Scotland, UK)

# Acknowledgements

The report is written in a group. In the national chapters, the national partners have worked with the literature, laws and codes in their own language area. This has meant collaboration with many people and the authors want to express their deepest gratitude for their help to following persons:

**FINLAND**
Mr D. Kivinen & R. Kurkijärvi; Transmasters Oy
S. Sierla, PhD Student & Professor R. Lahti; Faculty of Law, University of Helsinki
Mrs R. Kurki, Secretary
H. Tepponen, RN, MSc, PhD Student, T. Nyrhinen, RN, MSc, PhD Student,
M-L. Antila, RN, Master Student; University of Turku
P. Koskelainen, The Finnish Ministry of Social Affairs and Health, Kansainvälisten asioiden toimisto


**GERMANY**
M. Ulbricht, RN, Student
K. Klapper, RN, Student
S. Schulz-Ulricher, RN, Student
Humboldt-Universität


**GREECE**
A. Merkouris, MSc, PhD, RN, Evangelismos Hospital
A. Panagiotou, MSc, RN
M. Kapela, Graduate Student
M. Kalafati, Graduate student


**SPAIN**
J. Corbella, PhD, Lawyer, Legal Adviser in Law, Hospital de la Santa Creu in Sant Pau


**UNITED KINGDOM**
C. Dupuy, B.A., Edinburgh University
Cheryl Tringham, University of Stirling

# Contents

Authors    v
Acknowledgements    vi
Preface    ix
List of tables and figures    x

**Introduction**    1

**Chapter 1. Patient's autonomy, privacy and informed consent in legal norms and
professional codes**    5
1. General overview of the promotion of patients' rights    5
2. Legal norms in Finland, Germany, Greece, Spain and the United Kingdom    9
    2.1 Finland    9
    2.2 Germany    18
    2.3 Greece    25
    2.4 Spain    32
    2.5 The United Kingdom    36
3. Professional codes in health care in Finland, Germany, Greece, Spain, and the United
Kingdom    40
    3.1 General    40
    3.2 Finland    42
    3.3 Germany    44
    3.4 Greece    48
    3.5 Spain    50
    3.6 The United Kingdom    51

**Chapter 2. Patient's autonomy in the literature**    55
1. General    55
2. The concept of autonomy    56
3. Dimensions of the concept of autonomy    56
4. Realisation of autonomy    60
    4.1 Factors supporting autonomy    60
    4.2 Factors restricting autonomy    63
5. Autonomy in empirical studies    66
    5.1 General    66
    5.2 Autonomy and care of the elderly and chronically ill    67
    5.3 Autonomy and acute care    74
    5.4 Autonomy in gynaecological and maternity care    77

**Chapter 3. Patient's privacy in the literature**    79
1. General    79
2. The concept of privacy    80
    2.1 Perspectives in concept descriptions    81
    2.2 Dimensions of the concept of privacy    83
3. Realisation of privacy    90
    3.1 Factors supporting privacy    90

3.1 Factors supporting privacy                                          90
3.2 Factors restricting privacy                                         92
4. Privacy in empirical studies                                         94
    4.1 General                                                         94
    4.2 Privacy and care of the elderly and chronically ill            98
    4.3 Privacy and acute care                                         102
    4.4 Privacy in gynaecological and maternity care                   105

**Chapter 4. Informed consent in the literature**                      109
1. General                                                             109
2. The concept of informed consent                                     110
    2.1 Dimensions of the concept of informed consent                  112
3. Realisation of informed consent                                     114
    3.1 Factors supporting informed consent                            114
    3.2 Factors restricting informed consent                           117
4. Informed consent in empirical studies                               120
    4.1 General                                                         120
    4.2 Informed consent and care of the elderly and chronically ill   126
    4.3 Informed consent and acute care                                127
    4.4 Informed consent and gynaecological or maternity care          132

**Discussion and conclusions**                                         135

**References**                                                         139

# Preface

Questions of ethics have been attracting increasing attention in the health care debate during the past decade, not only in Europe but in other Western countries as well. There is accordingly a growing need for ethics research, which is further underlined by the fact that there is very little earlier work on everyday nursing procedures. The challenge concerns researchers working in all lines of inquiry in the field of health care: nursing researchers, medical doctors, ethicians and health economics researchers.

One of the most important areas of study in health care ethics is represented by the patient's status and rights. In the case of patient rights, key issues include patient autonomy, privacy and informed consent. These are the issues that are at the centre of attention here in this report. The present overview of the literature is intended to benefit various groups of health care professionals. The first of these groups is that of nursing and medical professionals: the aim is to increase their knowledge about legislation, ethical codes and research and in this way to support them in ethical decision-making. Secondly, the report provides useful material for people responsible for the design of ethics courses, which play a pivotal part in the education of ethically competent professionals. Thirdly, the report also serves the needs of researchers in search of new relevant research questions.

Health care clients are increasingly conscious about their rights and interested in the quality of health care services. It is reasonable to assume then that this overview also serves the interests of individual clients and patient organisations seeking answers to ethical questions. In particular, the report sheds light on the question of how patient rights materialise in everyday nursing situations: in situations where the clients' views really count, where they can take a meaningful part in the decision-making and which have a close bearing on their own everyday well-being.

This report has been written as part of the project on "Patients' autonomy, privacy and informed consent in nursing interventions", supported through the BIOMED2 programme by the European Commission. The project is scheduled to run for three years (1998-2001). The literature review was carried out in the first stage of the project, providing the groundwork for empirical data collection. Gathered in all five countries involved in the project, the purpose of the empirical material is to evaluate the realisation of autonomy, privacy and informed consent in surgical, maternity and long term elderly patients.

The following universities are involved in the project: the University of Turku (Finland), Humboldt Universität (Germany), the University of Athens (Greece), Escola Universitaria d'Infermeria, Hospital de la Santa Creu i Sant Pau (Spain) and the University of Stirling (UK). Project coordination is through the Department of Nursing at the University of Turku. All participating universities have contributed to the funding of the project. In addition, the Academy of Finland provided funding for the project in 1998-1999. Grant has also been obtained from the Finnish Nurses' Federation for a presentation at international congress.

We hope that this report will encourage readers to join in a more concerted effort to improve the ethical quality of health care.

December 29th 1999, Turku, Finland,

Helena Leino-Kilpi, Professor
Co-ordinator, scientist in charge

## LIST OF TABLES

Table 1.   Major declarations and conventions
Table 2.   Finnish Acts pertaining to patients' right to be informed
Table 3.   Summary of main laws related to autonomy, privacy and informed consent in Germany
Table 4.   Perspectives on the concept of autonomy
Table 5.   Categories of privacy in acute care setting
Table 6.   Definitions of informed consent
Table 7.   Prerequisites for informed consent

## LIST OF FIGURES

Figure 1.   Nursing interventions and ethics in health care
Figure 2.   Dimensions of the concept of autonomy
Figure 3.   Factors supporting autonomy
Figure 4.   Factors restricting autonomy
Figure 5.   Dimensions of the concept of privacy
Figure 6.   Factors supporting privacy
Figure 7.   Factors restricting privacy
Figure 8.   Basic dimensions of informed consent
Figure 9.   Factors supporting informed consent
Figure 10.  Factors restricting informed consent

# Introduction

The status and rights of patients have figured centrally in the debate that has been waged over the past two decades on questions of biomedical ethics (e.g. MacIntyre 1977, Pichler 1992, Leenen 1994, Westerhall & Phillips 1994, The Finnish Ministry of Social Affairs and Health 1996). The growing international attention is reflected in other documents "A Declaration on the Promotion of Patients' Rights in Europe", adopted in March 1994 by the World Health Organization (WHO 1994). Various non-governmental organisations have also advocated patients' rights and interests with a view to making these rights legally valid (Leenen 1994). A number of new laws on the status and rights of patients have been adopted in Europe, including Finland (Liljeström 1993, Kokkonen 1994, Lahti 1994, The Finnish Ministry of Social Affairs and Health 1996), Holland, Iceland and Lithuania (Nikkilä 1998). The importance of the patient-centred approach is also recognised in other aspects of health care (WHO 1998a,b), particularly in evaluations of the quality of care based on patient satisfaction surveys (Ross et al. 1987, Hall & Dornan 1988, Bond & Thomas 1992, Leino-Kilpi & Vuorenheimo 1992, Meisenheimer 1992, Leino-Kilpi & Kurittu 1995, Thomas & Bond 1996, WHO 1996a, O'Malley 1997, Merkouris et al. 1999a,b).

The biggest group of health care professionals in Europe is represented by nurses (WHO 1997). The aim of the nursing profession is to promote and support the health of clients, to strengthen their skills of self-care (e.g. Orem 1991), help them cope with their illness (e.g. Miller 1992) and support in dying (Henderson 1969). More broadly, nurses also have an obligation to promote the value of health in society (e.g. WHO 1993, Thompson et al. 1994, WHO 1994). All this means that nurses need to work very closely with their clients. They need to be highly qualified and base their work on nursing research and science. However, nursing research remains less developed in some European countries. Recognising this shortcoming, the Council of Europe (1996) has recently published a set of recommendations on how nursing research should be organised in Europe. Special emphasis is placed on raising the quality standards of nursing care and on assessing those standards by means of empirical research.

Nursing interventions are very common in everyday treatment and practice. Although these interventions can be described in different ways (e.g. Snyder 1985, Heater et al. 1988, Carpenito 1989, Leino-Kilpi 1990, Orem 1991, Bulechek & McCloskey 1992, Clark & Lang 1992, Saba 1995, Arndt 1998a), patient autonomy and privacy questions figure centrally in almost all of them. There has been no extensive and systematic research into the outcomes of nursing interventions (Abraham et al. 1995, Griffiths 1995), yet nursing literature point to obvious ethical problems relating to nursing interventions and patients autonomy and privacy (see Jecker 1991, Arndt 1994, Wainwright 1995). It has been found, for instance, that caregivers in nursing homes have difficulty providing patients with the opportunity to act autonomously (Ekman & Nordberg 1988) and that nurses tend to plan and implement interventions without asking patients what they think (Elander & Hermerén 1989).

Nursing occurs in a highly complex working environment which gives rise to varied and often intricate ethical problems (see Scott 1995, 1997, 1998). Many client groups such as elderly and dependent persons are also highly dependent on the care they receive (Dijkstra 1998). Some clients may also have difficulties exercising their autonomy on account of mental problems (Välimäki et al. 1996, Välimäki & Helenius 1996, Välimäki 1998). Furthermore, in the increasingly high tech environment that is the modern hospital, patients may be excluded from decision-making on their own care because the decisions may require specialised medical knowledge. A case in point is provided by surgical patient groups. On the other hand, some nursing/midwifery interventions have to do with natural life events such as childbirth. Still mothers do not necessarily have a say in how their childbirth is attended, the place of birth and in the interventions taking place (see e.g. Department of Health 1993, Crafter & Rowan 1998).

It is important not to address the question of patient autonomy from too narrow a perspective; several complex factors are involved that may influence the treatment of a patient. It is the duty of nursing staff to respect the patient's autonomy, but at the same time to act in the patient's best interests, and to prevent them from hurting themselves and others (Thompson et al. 1994, Bandman & Bandman 1995). It follows that staff are confronted by ethical conflicts every day which make it difficult for them to work in an autonomy-supporting manner. On the other hand, the meaning of the concepts of autonomy, privacy and informed consent are themselves highly complicated (Beauchamp & Childress 1994) and therefore difficult to implement in practice. Given all these conceptual, ethical and practical problems, how exactly can patients autonomy and privacy be supported (see Gadow 1989a,b, Yeo & Dalzier 1991, Bandman & Bandman 1995)?

The present report has been written in the context of the BIOMED2 project, Patient's Autonomy, Privacy, and Informed Consent in Nursing Interventions. The three-year project covers the period from 1998 to 2001 and is funded by the European Commission. It involves five European countries: Finland (University of Turku, Department of Nursing, coordinator), Germany (Humboldt Universität, Institut für Medizin-/Pflegepädagogik und Pflegewissenschaft), Greece (National and Kapodistrian University of Athens, Department of Nursing), Spain (Escola Universitaria d'Infermeria, Hospital de la Santa Creu i Sant Pau) and the United Kingdom, Scotland (University of Stirling, Department of Nursing and Midwifery). This report is the result of a joint effort of all these parties. It consists of a literature review produced by the five partners involved in the project; each partner is responsible for the national section they have written.

This report describes the contents of the three main concepts that are at the centre of attention in this project: patient autonomy, privacy and informed consent. The study focuses on three different groups: mothers with infants or babies in postnatal wards, surgical patients in hospital wards, and long-term elderly patients in institutions. These specific groups have been singled out for three reasons. Firstly, mothers who are having a baby represent a "healthy" group among nursing/midwifery clients. Delivery is considered a natural life event and the role of nurses and midwives is to support mothers to act independently with their baby. There are, however, some unique interventions such as informing mothers, helping them with their labour pains, and teaching them about breastfeeding and how to take care of their baby (WHO 1996b).

Secondly, surgical patients are included in the study because they represent a group whose body will be touched in a surgical operation and their physical integrity may be violated by health care personnel (see Burgoon 1982, Parrott et al. 1989). The purpose of nursing interventions is to help the patients recover after that operation. However, these patients are often in pain, they have many physiological symptoms, and they are in need of highly specialised technological interventions as well as interventions attending to their everyday physical needs.

Thirdly, we will be looking at the case of elderly patients in long-term care because they represent one particular stage of the life-span in which they show normal features of ageing. At the same time they may have several health problems. Failing to cope with activities of everyday living, this group of patients is often highly dependent on help from other people and they need advocates (see eg. Bandman & Bandman 1995). In addition, the nature of the support they receive is long-term. The role of nurses is therefore to understand the elderly patients ageing process, to support their orientation and activity in the environment and to help them to cope in their everyday life. In summary, then, we are chiefly interested in the key concepts of the ethics of professional caring manifest in nursing interventions as needed by different groups of people and in different life stages and situations. Our interest in nursing/midwifery interventions will be focused on nurses/midwives taking care of patient's diet, the administration of medication, patients' elimination and body hygiene. (Figure 1.) For reasons that have to do with language complications, the concept of nursing is used here in a broad sense as comprising midwifery interventions as well.

The overview is based primarily on the Medline and Cinahl-databases. Other sources include relevant legislation, professional codes, books and reports, whereas editorials, letters, comments or descriptions by special organisations are excluded. In spite of difficulties in gathering literature data in different countries we hope that this report provides a satisfactory overview of the area of literature related to patient autonomy, privacy and informed consent and that readers find the list of references useful. The rationale for the presentation of the report is simple. Firstly, the report attempts to increase health care professionals' knowledge of this problematic area. Secondly, it aims to support their ethical decision-making abilities, and thirdly it is to help health care educators and researchers to find the relevant literature in this area, and to provide information on what has already been studied in this area, and where the possible gaps lie.

The basic assumption in our report is that understanding consumers' and nurses' perceptions of patients' autonomy and privacy, as it applies to nursing interventions, will help to improve the ethical quality of care (see Meisenheimer 1992). The value of this report is further underscored by the fact that general ethical problems are often quite similar in different countries. However, as Quintana (1993) has observed, there are still important differences between European countries in terms of their national health care systems, the content of legislation and ethical codes concerning the status and rights of patients. Some ethical problems may also be experienced differently in different cultural contexts (see Tadd 1998). In the Nordic countries, for instance, respect for patient autonomy has a relatively long tradition, whereas in Mediterranean countries the family very often assumes responsibility for decision-making on behalf of the patient (Quintana

1993). It is therefore important to find out whether there is any evidence in the literature
to support this view.

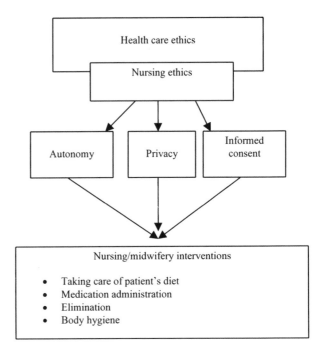

**Figure 1.** Nursing interventions and ethics in health care


       The report is structured around its four main content areas. Following this
introduction and a description of the literature used, the report moves on to describe
patient's autonomy, privacy and informed consent as they appear in the legal norms and
ethical codes. These concepts are discussed in separate chapters. Each chapter describes
the concept itself and how its content is understood through an overview of empirical
research in the relevant area. The report ends with a section on conclusions and a
discussion.

# Patient's autonomy, privacy and informed consent in legal norms and professional codes

## 1. General overview of the promotion of patients' rights

Laws and normative rules can have an important "push" effect, influencing and changing deep-rooted traditions in health care (WHO 1996a). In the area of patient autonomy, privacy and informed consent, the important norms are ones that have to do with patients' rights. Statements of rights provide protection of life, liberty, expression and property. They protect against oppression, unequal treatment, intolerance or arbitrary invasion of privacy (Beauchamp & Childress 1994).

However, the history of patients' rights is relatively short, beginning with the Universal Declaration of Human Rights in 1948 (Arndt 1996a). Declarations are statements of facts, of deeds done, care of actions taken. They are not laws, but they are firmer documents than codes. Declarations have taken on an air of solemnity, often of urgency, and for the most part, they contain statements of implied rights rather than rules of conduct. (Tschudin 1986, see Scheinin 1992.)

In this chapter, we begin by outlining the historical development of declarations and of legal and ethical norms related to the promotion of patients' rights. We then concentrate on the five European countries represented in this report, i.e. Finland, Germany, the Great Britain, Greece and Spain, and describe how patient autonomy, privacy and informed consent are endorsed in legal norms and ethical codes.

Patients' rights are a combination of legislation and principles, including ethical guidelines for different professional groups. Norms are also divided into legal and moral norms. The judicial part of the rights includes civil rights for patients and the duties of health care personnel. Patients' rights are based on general agreements, consensus and the will to uphold the principles agreed upon. (WHO 1996a.) The rights also have more general manifestations, for example as general human rights. By signing international declarations of human rights, states pledge to follow them in their own legal norms.

It is not possible to describe here all the declarations affecting the health care environment outlined in this report. Some of the major declarations are presented in Table 1. One significant turning point for patients' rights was the year 1947, when the Nüremberg Code was drawn up after revelations about Nazi war crimes. It was the first declaration on experimentation on human subjects (Massué 1998). This code was followed by one of the most commonly cited declarations, the Universal Declaration of Human Rights, adopted by UN General Assembly resolution of 10 December 1948. This declaration includes 30 articles concerning human rights. In addition, the International Codes of Medical Ethics describe the duties of physicians.

In today's Europe, a great deal of emphasis is placed on human rights. For example, membership of the Council of Europe is conditional on the Member State's ratification of the European Convention of Human Rights. This is based on Article 3 of the Statute of the Council of Europe on the principle of the rule of law, human rights and fundamental freedoms. In the context of the Council of Europe, the main instrument in the field on human rights is the European Convention for the Protection of Human Rights and Fundamental Freedoms, signed in Rome on 4 November 1950  (Arndt 1996a, Pellonpää 1996). The rights and fundamental freedoms guaranteed by the Convention are the right to life, the right to liberty and security of person; the right to fair trial in civil and criminal cases; the right to freedom of thought, conscience and religion; and the right of freedom of expression. (Tarschys 1998).

**Table 1.** Major declarations and conventions

| Declarations and conventions | Year |
|---|---|
| • The Universal Declaration of Human Rights | 1948 |
| • International Codes of Medical Ethics | 1949 |
| • Nüremberg Code | 1949 |
| • The European Convention for the Protection of Human Rights and Fundamental Freedom | 1950 |
| • The European Social Charter | 1961 |
| • Twelve Principles of Provisions of Health Care in Any Natural Health Care System | 1963 |
| • Declaration of Helsinki | 1964 |
| • International Covenant on Civil and Political Rights | 1966 |
| • Declaration of Sidney | 1968 |
| • Declaration of Geneva | 1968 |
| • Declaration of Oslo | 1970 |
| • Declaration of Tokyo | 1975 |
| • The Covenant on Economy, Social and Cultural Rights | 1976 |
| • Declaration of Lisbon | 1981 |
| • Declaration of Children's Rights | 1981 |
| • Declaration of Venice | 1983 |
| • Declaration of Euthanasia | 1987 |
| • Declaration of Lisbon | 1993 |
| • The Declaration of Promotion of Patients' Rights in Europe | 1994 |
| • The Convention for the Protection of Human Rights and Dignity of Human Being | 1997 |

In 1961, the European Social Charter was adopted of 18 October (1961). The rights and principles listed in the European Social Charter concern the protection of employment, including the following aspects:

- the right to work
- protection in the work environment
- the right to organise, the right to bargain collectively and the right of workers to information and consultation as well as the right to participate in the determination and improvement of the working conditions and working environment
- protection for certain categories of workers such as children and young persons, women, handicapped persons, and migrant workers.

Social protection for all of the population also includes the right to protection of health, the right to social security and the right to social and medical assistance, as well as the right to benefit from social welfare services. In addition, the Charter includes the right to special protection outside the work environment for children and young persons, mothers, families, handicapped persons, migrant workers and their families, and elderly persons. (The European Social Charter 1961.)

In 1963, Twelve Principles of Provisions of Health Care in Any National Health Care System were adopted by the 17th World Medical Assembly in New York (amended in 1983) (Hannikainen 1992). Another international covenant that has had an enormous impact in Europe is the International Covenant on Civil and Political Rights, adopted by UN General Assembly resolution of 16 December 1966, protecting traditional freedoms like the right to live and the right to personal freedom. The Covenant also states that no one shall be subjected to cruel, inhuman or degrading treatment or, without free consent, to medical or scientific experimentation. (Ilveskivi 1997a.)

The Declaration of Helsinki (1964, revised in Tokyo 1975, Venice 1983, Hong Kong 1989) was adopted by the text of the World Medical Association. The code of practice for Biomedical Research (Hannikainen 1992) gives recommendations to guide the physician (Massué 1998). It details the methods and conditions of experimentation, stipulating, in particular, that the association of research with care is justified only by diagnostic or therapeutic usefulness to the patient. It also affirms the primacy of the subject's welfare that overrides the interests of science and society. (Cüer 1998.) The Declaration includes four parts: introduction, basic principles, medical research combined with professional care, and non-therapeutic medical research involving human subjects.

The United Nations' International Covenant on Economic, Social and Cultural Rights, adopted by General Assembly resolution in 1966 (international entry into force in 1976), guarantees in its 12 articles the right of everyone to the enjoyment of the highest attainable standard of physical and mental health. This is a right for everybody, without discrimination of any kind as to race, colour, sex, language, religion, political or other opinion, national or social origin, property, birth or other status. (Ilveskivi 1997a.)

The Declaration of Sydney (1968) is a statement on the determination of death (Thompson et al. 1994). The Declaration of Geneva (1968) is the Code of the World Medical Association. It is shorter than the Hippocratic Oath that emphasises that the first consideration of the physician is the health of the patient (Downie & Calman 1994). The Declaration of Oslo (1970) is a statement on therapeutic abortion (Thompson et al. 1994). The Declaration of Tokyo (1975) gives guidelines for medical doctors, concerning torture and other cruel, inhuman or degrading treatment or punishment in the context of detention and imprisonment. In 1977, the World Psychiatric Association adopted the Hawaii Declaration. It is concern with psychiatric research and stresses the patient's freedom to withdraw consent to treatment or participation in a research programme for any reason and at any time (Massué 1998).

The EU's Directive (95/46/EU) is illustrative of the protection of individuals in the processing and free movement of personal data. Recommendations for the rights of hospital patients can also be found in a 1979 document of the European Economic Community Committee on Hospitals. A recommendation is not a legally-binding instrument, but it can have an effect on the interpretation of legally-binding norms. The declaration includes the following rights of hospital patients: the right to humanely administered, respectful and clinically appropriate treatment, the right to consent to care or refuse it, the right to know the risks in advance, the right to be afforded privacy, the right to have their religious and philosophical convictions respected and the right to complain. (Ilveskivi 1997a.)

The Declaration of Lisbon (1981, adopted in 1995) also focuses on patients' rights. Issues dealt with include the rights to freedom of choice and self-determination, the situation of the unconscious or legally incompetent patient, procedures against the patient's will, the right to information, the right to confidentiality, the right to health education, the right to dignity, and the right to religious assistance. The World Medical Association states that "a physician shall respect the rights of patients" (Anrys 1998). Furthermore, the Declaration on Euthanasia (1987) states that euthanasia is unethical, even at the patient's own request or at the request of close relatives.

Major international organisations have been involved in the development, promotion and implementation of patients' rights in Europe. These organisations include The Council of Europe, WHO, the World Medical Association and the European Union. (WHO 1996a.) The WHO Regional Office for Europe carried out a study in 1988-1989 on patients' rights in Europe. It clearly demonstrated the need to formulate a new declaration on patients' rights, taking into account the international human rights instruments and the conditions of and outlook for the practice of medicine. This problem was discussed at a European Consultation in Amsterdam from 28 to 30 March 1994. It resulted in "Declaration on the Promotion of Patients' Rights in Europe". (Rivero & Galán 1998.) The four main points of the Declaration, concerning patient autonomy, privacy and informed consent, are as follows:

- Human rights and values in health care: everyone has the right to be respected as a human being; the right to self-determination; to physical and mental integrity and to the security of his or her person; to have his or her privacy respected; to have his or her moral and cultural values and religious and philosophical convictions respected; and everyone have the right to the protection of health and to the opportunity to pursue his or her own highest attainable level of health.
- Information: the right to receive information about the availability of health services, about one's own condition and about applicable treatment, including information about the health care providers.
- Consent: the informed consent of the patient is a prerequisite for any medical intervention. A patient also has the right to refuse or to halt a medical intervention.
- Confidentiality and privacy: all information of a personal kind must be kept confidential. It can only be disclosed if the patient gives explicit consent or if the law expressly provides for this. There can be no intrusion into a patient's private and family life.

The treaties of the Council of Europe also include the Convention for the Protection of Human Rights and Dignity of the Human Being (1997). The purpose of this Convention is to protect the dignity and identity of all human beings and to guarantee everyone, without discrimination, respect for their integrity and other rights and fundamental freedoms with regard to the application of biology and medicine. It highlights, for example, the person's consent; private life and right to information; the human genome; scientific research; and organ and tissue removal from living donors for transplantation purposes.

In some countries, there are juridical norms governing patients' rights (Kokkonen 1994). The first countries to introduce such juridical norms were Spain (The General Health Act 1986), Finland (in 1993) and Holland (1995). In Israel, Lithuania and Iceland, laws governing patients' rights came into force in 1997. Some countries (e.g. the UK) have a so-called Patients' Charter, a declaration of patients' rights, or managed care contracts. These are not, however, juridically binding (Nikkilä 1998.)

The next few chapters describe the legal norms and charters that promote patients' rights, especially in Finland, Germany, Greece, Spain, and the United Kingdom.

## 2. Legal norms in Finland, Germany, Greece, Spain and the United Kingdom

*2.1 Finland*

In Finland, the status and rights of patients have been affected not only by legislation but also by conventional justice, regulations and guidelines of health care authorities, international human rights conventions and recommendations, and the ethical guidelines of the various groups of health care professionals. (Partanen 1993). However, the Constitution Act of Finland from 1919 did not expressly provide for the right to health and health care services, and the various statements of patients' rights were scattered in different laws.

Section 6 of the Constitution Act (Suomen Hallitusmuoto) speaks of the protection of life and personal freedom, which leads to the right to self-determination in matters concerning treatment. The section on freedom has been interpreted as implying the right to self-determination over one's own body. In practice, however, decisions involving the question of patients' rights could be based on a variety of sources, principles and rules of law or even norms that were not part of the judicial system. (see Ilveskivi 1997a.)

Although the important ideological point of departure in the improvement of the legal position of patients in Finland goes back to the 1960s (Lahti 1994), the status of human rights and fundamental rights in the judicial culture of Finland has really only been considerably strengthened during the 1990s, with the ratification of the European Convention of Human Rights (1990) and the reform of the Constitution Act in 1995 (Lahti 1997). At the end of the 1960s, the many different kinds of measures imposed upon an individual against his or her will were subjected to critical examination from the viewpoint of the civil rights of the individual concerned (Lahti 1994). The principle of self-determination was first validated in Finland in 1973 by the Parliamentary Ombudsman (Eduskunnan oikeusasiamiehen kertomus 1973).

Discussions about an explicit act on patients' status and rights started in the early 1980s. In 1980, the Commission on Legal Safeguards in Health and Medical Care, set up by the Ministry of Social Affairs and Health, proposed that a statutory patient insurance system should be adopted and a special law on the rights of patients ought to be enacted (Partanen 1993, Lahti 1994). Questions relating to patients' rights had to be clarified in a number of committees and reports. (Komiteamietintö 1982:65, STM 1986, see also Partanen 1993, Kokkonen 1994, Korhonen 1994, Lahti 1994). In 1991, the government introduced a bill to the Parliament (HE 1991), and the Act on the Status and Rights of Patients (Laki potilaan asemasta ja oikeuksista 785/92) came into force on 1 May 1993. Finland was thus the first country in Europe to implement an act on patients' rights. (Pahlman et al. 1996).

The Act on the Status and Rights of Patients (785/92) provides for the patient's right to good health care, medical care or related care when in need; the right of access to treatment, within resources; the right to be informed about treatment and care and the right to self-determination; the status of minor patients; emergency treatment; and the powers of the representative of the patient in certain situations. The law also established a complaint procedure and a patient ombudsman institution.

Today, there are several acts relating to patients' status and rights in Finnish legislation. One of the basic acts is the Act on Primary Health Care (Kansanterveyslaki 66/72). Together with the Act on the Status and Rights of Patients (785/92), it forms the legal basis for Finnish health care (Lahti 1997). The Act on Primary Health Care provides for services in all municipalities: e.g. health education, medical treatment, nursing care and rehabilitation, mental health services, transportation, dental care, school health care, student health care, occupational health care and screening. The act also stipulates that Finnish inhabitants must be able to use their mother tongue, be it either Finnish or Swedish.

The Patient Injury Act (Potilasvahinkolaki 585/86) brought major improvements to the status of patients. On the basis of this law, the patient will receive compensation for any injury to the person that occurs in connection with health care or medical treatment. Injury to the person is here taken to mean death, bodily harm, disease or illness (Lahti 1995). In order to improve the patient's indemnity protection, the Patient Injury Act introduced a statutory liability insurance system that was, in most cases, considered a fair substitute to conventional action to enforce indemnity liability and punitive damages (Lahti 1997).

The Act on Specialized Medical Care (Erikoissairaanhoitolaki 1062/89) governs specialist medical, dental and nursing care. Specialist care means health care services in some special field of medicine or odontology. The services can include prevention of illness, research, treatment, medical rescue operations or medicinal rehabilitation (1 §). According to this Act, patients should have the option of choosing which of the physicians in the hospital attends to them, within limitations set by the need to ensure efficient functioning of the hospital. Patients must be able to obtain services in their own language, whether it be Finnish or Swedish. The Act Concerning Health Care Professionals (Laki terveydenhuollon ammattihenkilöistä 559/94) seeks to promote patient security and the quality of health care services. The purpose of the Act is to guarantee that health care professionals have sufficient professional qualifications and the skills required to function in the profession.

Furthermore, the legal position of patients is touched upon in a number of special laws, such as the Mental Health Act (Mielenterveyslaki 1116/90), Act on Sterilization (Steriloimislaki 283/70), The Castration Act (Kastroimislaki 282/70), The Act on the Interruption of Pregnancy (Laki raskauden keskyttämisestä 239/70), The Act and Degree on National Personal Records Kept Under the Health Care System (Laki 556/89 ja asetus 774/89 Terveydenhuollon valtakunnallisista henkilörekistereistä), The Act on Social Work with Intoxicant Abusers (Päihdehuoltolaki 41/86), The Communicable Diseases Act (Tartuntatautilaki 583/86), and the Act on Special Care for the Retarded (Laki kehitysvammaisten erityishuollosta 519/77).

In 1995, a constitutional reform was implemented in Finland (969/95). The provisions on fundamental rights were comprehensively reformed. Traditional freedoms were extended and further defined in line with declarations of human rights. The constitution also came to include regulations on economic, cultural and social rights. The need for a constitutional reform sprang from an outdated constitutional system, the integration of Europe and the national identity of Finns. (Ilveskivi 1997a.)

We shall next describe patient autonomy, privacy and informed consent in Finnish legislation.

*Autonomy and self-determination*

The term autonomy is not used in Finnish health care legislation. The legal term in Finland is self-determination, and it can be found in two acts. The first is the Act on Status and Rights of Patients (785/92, Section 6 "Patients' right to self-determination"), stating that patient care must be planned in mutual understanding with the patient. If the patient refuses a certain treatment or measure, he/she is to be treated, within the range of possibility, in another medically acceptable way, which is to be planned in mutual understanding with the patient. However, neither Finnish legislation in general nor The Act on Patients Status and Rights (785/92) gives a clear definition of treatment or the kind of situation where the patient's consent is required (Nikkilä 1998).

There are limitations to the self-determination of patients. According to Section 6 (785/92), if an adult patient, because of mental disturbance or mental retardation or for other reasons, is incapable of deciding about the treatment given to him/her, the legal representative or next of kin or other person close to the patient must be heard before important decisions concerning treatment can be made. This is done in order to assess what kind of treatment would be in accordance with the patient's wishes. If no such assessment can be made, the patient must be given treatment that can be considered to be in accordance with his/her best interest. Provisions on treatment given irrespective of the wishes of the patient are included in the Mental Health Act (1116/90), The Act on Social Work with Intoxicant Abusers (41/86), The Communicable Diseases Act (583/86), and in the Act on Special Care for the Retarded (517/77).

The second act governing self-determination is the Mental Health Act (1116/90) that discusses limitations to the right of self-determination (28 §). The right of self-determination of a person admitted for observation or referred for treatment may be limited, and coercive measures may be used only to the extent necessary for the treatment, for the patient's own safety or for the safety of others. The chief physician of the hospital or other physician in charge has the right to examine letters or parcels to a person who is under observation or who has been referred for coercive treatment or to be examined or withheld, if considered necessary in the interests of maintaining order or safety or if there are reasonable grounds to suspect that the letter or parcel contains intoxicant drugs. However, mail from the authorities overseeing the work of the hospital, judicial authorities or a legal advisor to the person under observation or referred for treatment must be delivered immediately without examination.

The Act on the Status and Rights of Patients (785/92) lists the measures to be taken when an adult patient, because of mental disturbance or mental retardation or for other reasons, is incapable of deciding about the treatment given to him/her (see above). The rights of incompetent patients are also discussed in The Act on Sterilization (283/70). Furthermore, according to The Act on the Interruption of Pregnancy (239/70), if a woman is incapable of making a competent request for pregnancy termination, due to mental illness, deficiency or disorder, and if there are pressing reasons for the pregnancy termination, the procedure can be carried out with the consent of the guardian or a specially appointed trustee.

The status of minor patients is discussed in Act (785/92), Section 7. According to the law, the minor patient's opinion on a treatment measure must be taken into account if the patient's age or level of development makes him/her capable of deciding about the treatment given to him/her. If the minor patient is of sufficient age or level of development, treatment must be planned in mutual understanding with him/her. If the minor patient is incapable of deciding about the treatment given to him/her, treatment is to be planned in mutual understanding with his/her guardian or legal representative.

Finnish law does not accept discrimination in health care. According to the Act on Status and Rights of Patients (785/92), any person residing permanently in Finland is entitled to health care and medical care, according to his/her health, without discrimination and within resources available to health care at the time in question. The patient has the right to health care and medical care of good quality. (Chapter 2, Section 3.) A patient who is not satisfied with the health care or medical care or treatment received has the right to make a complaint to the director responsible for health care. Making a complaint does not affect the patient's right to complain to health care authorities or medical care authorities about the care or treatment received. (Section 10.)

According to Section 11, a patient ombudsman shall be appointed for health care units. The tasks of the patient ombudsman are to advise patients as regards the application of this Act, to help patients with their complaints, to inform patients of their rights, and to act for the promotion and implementation of patients' rights.

*Privacy and confidentiality*

Confidentiality is one of the key principles of health care, and one that can be viewed from two angles: that of the patient and that of the functioning of health care. Patients have a right to expect that no outsider will come to obtain the information that they have provided or that has been otherwise acquired. Confidentiality in a doctor-patient relationship also presupposes protection of privacy (Ilveskivi 1997a.) However, the concept of protection of privacy is not easily defined. The protection of privacy has been considered e.g. in the draft bill for Personal Data File Act (HE 1986). According to the bill, protection of privacy can cover much more than just the private life of a person: except under certain special circumstances, the person does not have to impart personal information to the authorities unless the law expressly requires this.

Chapter II of the Council of Europe Convention for the Protection of Individuals with regard to Automatic Processing of Personal Data (European Treaty Series No. 108) which was opened for signature on 28 January 1981 (SopS 35/ and 36/92) documents the principles of protection of personal data. In Finland, the Convention came into force on 1 April 1992. Article 1 states that the Convention set out to maintain a "just balance between the different rights and interests of individuals" and in particular between the freedom to process information on the one hand and rights of privacy on the other. At the same time, Article 6 forbids the automatic processing of information relating to a person's health unless national legislation provides sufficient protection. (Ilveskivi 1997a,b.)

Patients' right to privacy is mentioned in the Act on Status and Rights of Patients (785/92), Section 3. According to the Act, the care and treatment of the patient must be such that the patient's human dignity is not violated and that his/her convictions and privacy are respected. The Act (Section 13) also states that information in patient documents is confidential. Health care professionals or other persons working in a health care unit or carrying out its tasks shall not give patient information to outsiders without written consent of the patient. The confidentiality rule continues to apply even after termination of the employment relationship or the task. However, there are some exceptions:

- Information may be given from patient documents to a court, another authority or community which by virtue of law is entitled to receive the information;
- Information necessary for the arrangement of examination and treatment may be given to another health care unit or health care professional in accordance with the patient's orally given consent or his/her consent that is otherwise obvious from the context;
- Information about the identity and state of health of the patient may be given to a member of the patient's family or an individual with whom the patient has a close personal relationship, if the patient receiving treatment is in a state of unconsciousness or other comparable state and if there is no reason to believe that the patient would object.

A variety of other Finnish acts touch on issues relating to confidentiality. The Act on the University of Helsinki Central Hospital (1064/89, 19 §) states that the provisions of Act on the Specialized Medical Care (1062/89, 57 §) apply. According to these provisions, elected officials of the hospital district of the federation of municipalities or other persons employed by, in the service of, or working in the hospital district may not, unless given consent, impart personal or family secrets that have come to their knowledge by virtue of their position or function. The confidentiality rule continues to apply even after termination of employment.

The Private Health Care Act (Laki yksityisestä terveydenhuollosta 152/92) states that an official who, while performing such duties as are prescribed in the Act, has received information about a trade secret or professional secret or the economic situation of the health care provider or about the personal circumstances of a person may not disclose this information without the consent of the person protected by the confidentiality rule (15 §, also The Act on Sterilization 283/70, 9 §).

At the same time, according to The Occupational Health Care Act (Työterveyshuoltolaki 743/78), the employer, occupational safety committee of the work place and the occupational safety officer are entitled to obtain, from persons working in occupational health service, such information as affects the health of the employees and the development of a healthier working environment, even though the information has come to the health care workers by virtue of their position. Information that is deemed confidential may not be disclosed without the consent of the person protected by the confidentiality rule. (6 §.)

As far as harmonisation of data protection and security in the area of health care records is concerned, the great leap forward has been the implementation of the Act on Status and Rights of Patients (785/92), while the main principles of data security have been based on the Personal Data File Act (471/86) and the Decree on Personal Data Register (476/87). Their provisions apply to the collecting, recording, using, delivering and archiving of data. They are also the source of the obligation to provide treatment and the security duty of the controller of the file, and giving details for the protection of the data. However, on June 1, 1999 a new Personal Data Act (532/99) entered into force with the purpose of promoting, firstly, the protection of privacy and other related basic rights in connection with the processing of personal data and, secondly the development of and compliance with good data security procedures (1 §).

Legislation that warrants attention also includes the Act on Public Document (83/51) which makes statements about researchers' access to patient information. It also makes special provisions for the transfer of data included in welfare and health legislation and the administrative decisions in these fields (Tervo-Pellikka 1994). Furthermore, The Act on National Personal Records Kept Under the Health Care System (Laki terveydenhuollon valtakunnallisista henkilörekistereistä 556/89 and rekisterien tietosisällöstä annettu asetus 774/89) are concerned with the confidentiality of information, while The Communicable Diseases Act (538/86, pykälä 23a) has information about a national register of communicable diseases, maintained by the National Public Health Institute. (Tanttinen & Rasimus 1994). Taking as the basis Section 5.3 in the Act on the Status and Rights of Patients (785/92) on the right to check data on oneself in patient documents. There are strict instructions for the procedure of correcting patient documents. (Tervo-Pellikka 1993.)

*Informed consent*

The principle of self-determination is illustrated by the fact that care is only permissible after consent has been given. This is the definition of the principle of informed consent. (Ilveskivi 1997a.) According to Kokkonen (1993), the principle of informed consent could be seen to inspire particular respect in Finland, considering that the Helsinki Declaration was born in the Finnish capital.

During the past two decades, patient consent has been discussed extensively in Finland, and especially in the following areas: clinical trials on drugs, patient's status in teaching, legislation on patients' rights, guidelines on terminal care, and the right of a Jehovah's witness to refuse blood transfusion. Furthermore, there has been discussion on the use of foetal tissue from aborted foetuses, on guidelines on medical research, living wills, a minor's consent, research concerning documents, and communication between doctors and patients. (Kokkonen 1993.) Informed consent can be divided into information and consent, where the information part covers both access to information and the capability to understand that information (Nikkilä 1998).

The patient's right to be informed is governed by several different norms at several different levels (Ilveskivi 1997b). One of the key norms is the Act on Status and Rights of Patients (785/92, Section 5), which expressly provides for the patient's right to be informed and also regulates it. According to the act, the patient shall be informed about his/her state of health and given a clear explanation of the treatment proposed. In addition, the patient has the right to know about appropriate alternative forms of treatment, their effects and any other factors, associated with the forms of treatment, that may have significance when decisions are made on the treatment. However, this information shall not be given against the will of the patient or when it is obvious that giving information would cause serious hazards to the life or health of the patient. Special regulations pertaining to the right to be informed can be found in a number of laws (Table 2).

**Table 2.** Finnish Acts pertaining to patients' right to be informed

| Acts | |
|---|---|
| The Act on the Interruption of Pregnancy | 239/70 |
| The Castration Act | 282/70 |
| The Act on Sterilization | 283/70 |
| The Act on Special Care for the Retarded | 519/77 |
| The Act on the Removal of Human Organs and Tissues For Medical Use | 355/85 |
| The Act on Social Work with Intoxicant Abusers | 41/86 |
| The Communicable Diseases Acts | 583/86 |
| The Mental Health Act | 1116/90 |
| The Act on Patient's Status and Rights | 785/92 |

As regards understanding the information received, health care professionals should try to give the information in such a way that the patient would be able to understand it to the extent necessary. If the health care professional does not know the language used by the patient or if the patient, because of a sensory handicap or speech defect, cannot be understood, interpretation should be provided if possible. (Act 785/92, Section 5.)

As for the requirement of informed consent, sections 5 – 9 of the Act (785/92) provide the most relevant information. In these sections, there are two important points that bring clarification and also a slight change in comparison with what used to be the common legal opinion. Firstly, sections 7 and 9 stipulate that if a minor patient is capable of deciding on the treatment given to him/her (i.e. understands the treatment), only the patient himself/herself can give valid consent and decide on the disclosure of information pertaining to his/her health and care. Secondly, section 8 prescribes that if the patient already has, steadfastly and competently, expressed his/her will concerning treatment given to him/her, he/she must not be given an emergency treatment either when he/she is actually incompetent because of unconsciousness or another reason. (Lahti 1994.)

Care of the patient has to be planned in mutual understanding with him/her. Act 785/92, Section 6 stipulates that, in the case of patient refusal, the patient has to be treated, within the range of possibility, in some other medically acceptable way selected in mutual understanding with the patient. According to the Act, if an adult patient, because of mental disturbance or mental retardation or for other reasons, is incapable of deciding about the treatment given to him/her, the legal representative or next of kin or other person close to the patient must be heard before important decisions concerning treatment can be made. This is done in order to assess what kind of treatment would be in accordance with the patient's wishes. If no such assessment can be made, the patient must be given treatment that can be considered to be in accordance with his/her best interests.

It has been stated that it is admissible to depart from the principle of consent in the case of just a small treatment. Asking for the patient's consent is not considered necessary if the treatment is considered insignificant or just a small part of the procedure; the fact that the patient has sought treatment is considered tacit consent where small treatments are concerned, especially if the treatments are necessitated by the patient's condition. However, it is impossible to formulate a general rule that would define "just a small treatment" for which the patient's consent were not required. It is, therefore, necessary to ascertain that the patient's wishes are known every time in unclear cases, and particularly if the treatment involves risks or if there are alternative methods of treatment available. The more seriously the health care personnel must impose upon the patient's bodily integrity, the more crucial it becomes to make sure that the patient's wishes are known. (HE 185/1991).

The draft bill examined in the above paragraph (HE 185/1991) also touches upon the form that the patient's consent should take. It is commonly thought that oral consent is sufficient when patients are asked about their wishes. Written consent is necessary if there is reason to believe that evidence of the consent will be needed at a later date. Finally, informed consent cannot be required in a situation where the patient does not want to be informed or refuses to receive the information. (HE 185/1991.)

*Some critique on acts relating to patients' rights in Finland*

The implementation of the Act on Status and Rights of Patients (785/92) has already been evaluated in Finland. Pahlman et al. (1996) describe experiences during the first three years of the Act being in force. The data were collected both by questionnaires from patient ombudsmen (N = 28) and by reviewing the complaints decided by Provincial Governments, from the beginning of 1995 to August 1995, and by the National Board of Medicolegal Affairs, in 1993 – 1995. According to the authors, the law has influenced practices within health care. Firstly, living wills have become more common as a manifestation of people's willingness to use their right to self-determination even when they are no longer able to express their wishes. Secondly, there are frequent complaints to be processed at the local level. Thirdly, every organisation today has a patient ombudsman. As a result of these developments, the principles of the system of patient ombudsmen and patients' right to complain have been evaluated as good, although there is still room for improvement. However, there is much to be improved in patients' access to information and in getting the nursing staff to encounter the patients as fellow humans. The authors argue that attitudes and health care traditions have changed slowly.

Some criticism has also been levelled at the acts relating to patients' rights. According to Lahti (1994), the requirement of informed consent itself has not been explicitly defined, and the form of consent is left open. Another major problem, is caused by the fact that the law has been written from the point of view of the rights of patients. As a consequence, implementation and sanctioning issues have not been addressed; questions of implementation and sanctioning tend to be decided on the basis of available resources, other health legislation and legal order in general. In a situation like this, there is always the risk of the law failing and becoming a mere symbolic piece of legislation.

In 1997, The Finnish Ministry of Social Affairs and Health (Sosiaali- ja terveysministeriö) established a development project, part of which involves making suggestions for the improvement of the status of patients in Finland, on the basis of national and Nordic data. On the one hand, it appears that the status of patients in Finland is secure and relatively well organised. Patients' rights are included in the law, and health care professionals are well educated. On the other hand, Finland does not have a strong culture of participation and the people are unaccustomed to using their influence. For example, patients seldom have the opportunity to choose the physician attending to them or the time and place of their treatment. There are also problems with the implementation of patients' rights. One statement in the project report suggests that the role of ombudsmen, in particular, should be clarified, and the manner in which patients are treated, given information and encouraged to use their right of self-determination should be improved. Another major problem was the lack of a national ethical board for health care. (Nikkilä 1998.) Further, although Finland has succeeded in introducing various safeguards for ordinary patients, few provisions govern medical research and the status and rights of research subjects at present (Lötjönen 1998).

In 1998, the Act on Status and Rights of Patients (785/92) was changed: the Council of State appointed a national ethical board of health care to function within the Ministry. The task of this board is to examine ethical questions and principles that relate to health care and the status of patients, and to issue recommendations. The composition and functions of the advisory committee are described more fully in the Act on the Amendment of the Act on Status and Rights of Patients (Laki potilaan asemasta ja oikeuksista annetun lain muuttamisesta 333/1998). The Act has additionally been criticised for being overly strict on data protection. This may prove a disadvantage e.g. in providing further care. If a patient dies without having given written consent to the care providers, no information about the patient can be disclosed; this confidentiality of information applies even when family members request information. (Pahlman et al. 1996.)

## 2.2 Germany

In the German literature issues of patient autonomy are primarily discussed from a medical and legal point of view, though also to some extent from a philosophical and theological angle. The views of nursing staff, however, are conspicuous in their absence: although nursing staff may be mentioned in the titles, they hardly appear in the texts at all (cf. Kollwitz 1997). In particular the issue of 'Truth at the bedside' has been discussed by doctors, lawyers and theologians for decades without giving vent to the dilemma as it applies to nursing staff (Hofmann 1996, 21).

Given the subordinate position of nursing staff to medical doctors in the health care hierarchy, it seems to be taken more or less for granted that nurses should also subordinate their conscience to the legal doctrine, without any consideration for ethical concerns (Hofmann 1996). It may often be nursing staff who actually have to carry out doctors' decisions and subsequent orders regarding patients in conditions such as persistent vegetative state as Richardson and Webber (1998) point out. Nurses may be asked to reduce care for particular patients, to remove a feeding tube, or to switch off a respirator. However, patients and their next of kin will usually show greatest confidence precisely in the nursing staff.

On the other hand, professional experience suggests that nursing staff often decline to answer patients' questions and fail to recognise their fundamental ethical responsibility. They deny their decision-making competencies, taking recourses to their incompetence in medical matters. This becomes evident in a study published by Arndt in 1997a. According to Ulfig (1997) the 'good life' as a prima facie moral notion depends on action on the basis of reason. Reason, that is, as informed by knowledge. If applied to nursing it becomes evident that appropriate knowledge must provide the basis of good care. If such knowledge does not exist nursing staff are doomed to remain silent and passive. Nurses must have knowledge of the different theories and technical terms and also establish their own assured position to be able to make a crucial contribution to ethical debates (Johnstone 1998).

In philosophy, autonomy is based on the abolition of heteronomy. The emphasis is on the possibility of free action by the autonomous subject, on the subject's ability to exercise reason and to decide on his or her own laws, norms and rules of action (Meyers grosses Taschenlexikon 1992). This conception can be traced back to Kantian ethics. Kant explains that in human beings, self-determination is only possible if they dissociate themselves from the direct influences of sensual impulses, desires, passions and interests if they free themselves from such heteronomy.

The superior ability of will (also called freedom of will) is realized if conformity to the law of one's own rule of action becomes the purpose of action. The ensuing consequence is that personal choice has to be based on a person's will informed by reason. According to Kant, autonomy is the highest principle of morality: "*Autonomy of the will is the sole principle of all moral laws and duties*" (Theorem 4, 1997, 30).

The individual commits him-/herself to determine the moral laws of his/her action on the basis of pure reason. The morally acting individual accepts the moral law he has chosen as universally binding; in every comparable situation, every other rational being will have to come to the same conclusion (categorical imperative) (see Ulfig 1997).

The relationship between the patient and doctor has been quite profoundly changed by the medical revolution as well as by developments in modern society at large. Medicine and medical treatment was traditionally bound by the Hippocratic oath, which requires that everything is done in the patients' best interests without doing any harm to them (Leist 1994, Schwerdt 1998). It follows that doctors focus their attention accordingly; the patient's will is not their primary concern (Vollmann 1997). Patients, for their part, have learned to trust the medical doctor's skills and abilities to guarantee their well-being (Körner 1994). This asymmetry between doctors and laypeople with respect to medical knowledge and skills contributes to paternalism and to paternalistic behaviour on the part of doctors towards patients (Kollwitz 1997).

In contrast, the emphasis today is on patient autonomy, giving patients the opportunity to choose the treatment they consider appropriate on the basis of their own value judgements at least theoretically. In modern medicine, patient autonomy is considered a necessary precondition, whereas previously it was considered superfluous and absurd. In Nazi-Germany medical doctors and other scientists as well as health care staff had killed and horrendously abused human beings in the name of social progress and in the name of medical science. After the second world war new emphasis was placed worldwide upon the Human Rights idea and the new German preliminary constitution of 1949 was based upon the principle of the inviolation of human dignity. (see Körner 1994.)

*The consequences of the German Constitution*

In Germany, the right to autonomy is based on Article 2 of the constitutional law set down in the Constitution (also Grundgesetz, Böhme 1991).
German Constitution, Article 2 (Rights of liberty):
▪ Everyone shall have the right to free development of his personality in so far as he does not violate the rights of others or offend against the constitutional order or the moral code.
▪ Everyone shall have the right to life and to inviolability of his person. The liberty of the individual shall be inviolable. These rights may only be encroached upon pursuant to a law.
This Article establishes the basis for the interpretation of the most important constitutional right, as laid down in Article 1: "The dignity of man shall be inviolable" (The Constitution, Article 1).

The contemporary understanding is that the constitutional rights in the Constitution are in principle universally binding, and not only with respect to the relationship between citizen and state ("third-party effect"). Legislation, executive power and jurisdiction are bound by the constitutional rights. The constitutional rights are worded in very general terms and therefore call for some explanation. For instance, there is no concrete definition of humane nursing in relation to "Pflegeversicherung" (compulsory care insurance in Germany; social security code XI § 11 Section 1) (cf. Sperl 1996), but this concept had to be derived from the human rights guaranteed through the Constitution.

Concrete declarations are set out in the social security code or arise from interpretations of the law in the case of rulings by the Supreme Court. The Federal Supreme Court declares that a doctor's obligation to heal the sick and to preserve life is limited by the individual's fundamentally free right of self-determination over his/her body (Böhme 1991). With only few exceptions, involuntary treatment is strictly prohibited (Brenner 1997). If a patient possessing all his or her faculties decides to refuse treatment, all medical and nursing interventions (help with feeding, medication) must be immediately discontinued (Brenner 1997, see also Böhme 1991). One important exception is the failure to help in suicide cases.

*Autonomy and personal liberty*

Personal freedom of movement is protected by the German Criminal Code § 239. Unlawful restriction of a person or the deprivation of a person's liberty carries the punishment of up to five years' imprisonment or a fine (Section 1). In case of wrongful deprivation of personal liberty lasting more than one week, the sentence is one to ten years' imprisonment (Section 2).

Deprivation of liberty is regulated by Article 104 of the Constitution. This Article includes the legal guarantee that individual freedom may only be restricted by virtue of a formal law, and states that detained persons must not be subjected to mental or physical ill-treatment.

Confinement to psychiatric clinics is regulated by federal laws of accommodation. The restrictions of liberty which require approval by a legal representative or guardian also include the containment of patients by means of belts or similar aids (Markus 1996a). Immobilisation may be permissible for short periods of time if there is the risk that the patient may put him- or herself or other people in danger. For instance, restraining an acutely disturbed mental patient for a short period of time would be justified on doctors orders only.

According to Böhme (1991), there are only a few exceptions where involuntary treatment may be considered:

- In cases of venereal disease (lues, gonorrhoea, ulcus molle, i. e. venereal inflammation of the lymph node), the patient is obliged to receive treatment until the risk of infection is over.
- In cases of cholera, typhus, plague and smallpox, the law says that hospital isolation is required. If the person concerned refuses, a district judge may order that person to be detained.

- In cases of serious danger to health, life-threatening dangers, or danger to the health of others, prisoners are subject to involuntary medical examination and treatment as well as forced feeding (Penal Law § 101).
- In cases where a mentally ill offender cannot be punished on grounds of diminished responsibility, it is possible to confine this person to a psychiatric clinic or borstal (Penal Law § 63 and § 64).
- Suspected offenders may be subjected to a physical examination for instance to have a blood test in order to ascertain facts crucial to criminal proceedings (Crimininal Code § 81).
- On certain conditions, for instance when they present a threat to their own lives or the lives of others, mentally ill persons may be subjected to compulsory accommodation and treatment in psychiatric hospitals. This is regulated by federal laws.
- Persons placed under guardianship (who were formerly called incapacitated persons) and wards may be accommodated on certain conditions, after approval has been sought by a guardian or "Rechtspfleger" (officials with certain administrative and judicial powers).

*Privacy and confidentiality*

The protection of a person's privacy is based on the constitutional rights of human dignity and free development of personality. The Federal Constitutional Court has coined the concept of the right to informational self-determination (1991), which means that personal data such as address, profession or denomination shall always be protected and must not be made available to third persons.

Physicians, nursing staff and certain other groups are under obligation not to divulge secret information that comes to their knowledge through the pursuance of their profession (Böhme 1991). Any violation of this obligation (according to Criminal Code § 203) may lead to imprisonment of up to one year or a fine. The secrecy obligation applies even in situations where a person representing the occupational groups concerned is called upon to make a statement in criminal or civil action (§ 52 ff. code for criminal procedures; § 383 ff. civil procedures).

The secrecy obligation also applies to the fact that a patient has been admitted to hospital. If a nurse divulges information to a stranger about a patient's health over the telephone, that also constitutes a violation, unless of course the nurse has the patient's consent to do so. This consent may also be given indirectly, for instance if a patient in a room with several beds mentions a problem on his/her own initiative in the presence of other patients (Böhme 1991). For the nursing staff, the legal situation means that they have to be extremely sensitive in dealing with information and even ask the patient's permission to put up personal data on the bed, for instance. As a matter of principle, no patient information should be released to outsiders. However, if the patient releases the nursing staff from the requirement of confidentiality, for instance towards his/her partner, then the nurse is allowed to give that information (Böhme 1991).

The duty to maintain confidentiality about personal data also applies to hospital management and other departments that are not directly involved in the patient's treatment.

In the case of young persons who are not old enough to give consent to a medical intervention, confidentiality must also be maintained towards their parents or legal guardians (Böhme 1991).

There are, however, certain exceptions to these security considerations. Social security institutions have the right to receive information on the patient (cf. e.g. German National Insurance Code § 1543). In the case of inquiries from health insurance institutions, professional associations and social insurance boards, health care staff are under no duty to maintain confidentiality because employees in these public institutions are also subject to confidentiality (Criminal Code § 203 II No. 2). In the case of children up to the age of fourteen, there is no duty to maintain confidentiality towards their parents or legal guardians (Böhme 1991).

The protection of privacy in the sense of data security also extends to correspondence (Criminal Code § 202, Section 1 No. 1): anyone who opens a sealed letter or document that is not intended for them and who has no authorisation to do so, is liable to punishment.

*Informed consent*

Based on European Enlightenment, the legal theory of informed consent was developed in the United States (Helmchen 1997). The requirement of consent ensues from Articles 1 and 2 of the German Constitution (Brenner 1997). In principle, any curative intervention entails bodily harm (Criminal Code § 223, § 224) (Böhme 1991) and therefore requires justification. The action is justified by the patient's consent (Criminal Code § 226), presumed consent, self-defence and necessity (Brenner 1997). Patient consent requires that this person has sufficient information about the significance and consequences of the medical intervention (cf. Federal Supreme Court judgements that establish a principle, in Böhme 1991). For this consent to have legal validity, the patient must also understand the information. In practice, however, it is often very difficult to meet this requirement (cf. Kranich 1997). Information on diagnosis and treatment is the sole responsibility of the consulting doctor (Böhme 1991). Mentally ill patients, minors and old people also have to be appropriately informed. This means that even in cases of accommodation for treatment which involves considerable risk for life or health, it is necessary to have the consent of the person concerned (e. g. for operations, electroconvulsive therapy).

German law also includes sections concerning the individual's incapacity. No conclusions can be drawn with respect to the person's capacity to consent on the basis of medical diagnosis alone (Vollmann 1997). The assessment of the capacity to consent is the responsibility of the medical profession, and is based not on legal competence but on the capacity to comprehend (Böhme 1991). In the case of inability to consent, it is required that the consent of the legal representative or guardian is obtained (Markus 1996a,b). A court application has to be made by a medical doctor in order to obtain guardianship for a patient (see Böhme 1991). The nursing literature on legal issues points clearly to the medical doctor's dominant role in such cases. Furthermore, medical doctor's legal responsibilities regarding treatment and hospital care provides nurses with a certain legal protection at the cost of reduced responsibility. It does not however, remove nurses' vicarious liability for nursing actions.

Apart from information on medical interventions (i.e. on self-determination), there is also the question of information on the diagnosis and on safety (Böhme 1991, Graw 1995). Information on the diagnosis involves the question as to whether the doctor is obliged to reveal his or her diagnosis to the patient. By and large the same aspects are relevant as in the case of informing on self-determination. Information on safety applies to the doctor's obligation to provide for the welfare of his or her patients for instance in terms of insurance law.

As far as medical interventions are concerned, the nursing staff have no own informational rights (Böhme 1991). Since both diagnosis and therapy are the sole responsibility of the physician, it follows that nursing staff have no obligation to inform the patient. According to Böhme (1991), the general task of informing cannot be delegated to the nursing staff. However, in specific cases it is possible to trust the relevant nurse with the responsibility of explaining and clarifying something to the patient, once the doctor has provided the basic information with respect to the intervention. In instances where the patient does not have all the necessary information, the nursing staff are not allowed to intervene, but they have to remind the doctor about his or her informational duties. This has to be done through official channels, i.e. through the director of nursing and the senior consultant or superintendent.

In the treatment of terminally ill patients, though, the nursing staff cannot be expected to conceal the truth indefinitely. The present monopoly of the medical profession in terms of the right to inform patients as to their condition and prognosis cannot be upheld. Ultimately nursing staff will have to be involved and legislation may well make provision for this (Böhme 1991, Arndt 1997a).

There is no legal duty to carry out medical and nursing interventions if patients who are in full possession of their faculties refuse to give their consent. This also applies to situations where the patient refuses without obvious reason to take the medication prescribed or to eat. In such cases, Brenner (1997, 28) says, "doctors and nursing staff cannot be punished for negligence (e.g. duty of care) according to Criminal Code § 323". Further, if a patient refuses an intervention that is deemed absolutely essential (such as taking medicine), the nurse is required to inform the doctor, who then has to decide whether the patient concerned is incapable to consent, and whether the patient's health or life are at risk. Finally, the nursing staff may and should disregard the patient's will only if no doctor is available and the patient's life is at risk (Böhme 1991).

For personal protection, it is recommended that nursing staff should record their interventions witnessed colleague (Böhme 1991). This is also recommended when restraining safety measures are applied, such as the use of bed rails without the patient's consent. However, in situations where a patient's safety is at risk nursing staff must seek doctor's orders if any form of restraint is to be used bar emergency situations (see Markus 1996a).

An intervention made without the patient's consent (for instance in cases of unconsciousness) is justified if the patient's health is acutely at risk and if there was no earlier opportunity to ask for the patient's consent (Civil Code § 677). Even if a relative is present and refuses to give consent, the principle of presumed consent applies (Böhme 1991).

Next of kin are not automatically taken as the patient's legal representatives, and consequently doctors are not legally bound by their will (Böhme 1991). This applies not only to euthanasia, but also for instance to confinement to a psychiatric hospital or measures of physical restraint. However, a relative may be appointed guardian, either in advance by the patient him-/herself or, in an acute situation, by a court of guardianship.

The principle of presumed consent is not applied if the patient has advanced a written statement of his or her decision. In practice, this means that the refusal of a Jehovah's Witness to have a blood transfusion will be accepted (Böhme 1991). The actual observance and application of patients' instruction (living will) with regard to treatment decisions has not yet been codified by law in Germany (Richter et al. 1998). It is doubtful whether the patient's will as set out in written instructions will be accepted as legally binding (Böhme 1991). This means the doctor will have some freedom of movement until the patient's condition allows for the ending of treatment on the basis of an unfavourable prognosis. Comparative cultural studies have shown that nursing staff tend to accept patients' directives more readily than do medical doctors (Richter et al. 1998). In cases where a diagnosis of persistent vegetative state has been established, after due considerations involving all people concerned with the case - including the wishes of the patient or the presumed wishes of the patient - there is no legal obligation for doctors to continue with treatment. The doctor's decision to discontinue treatment must not be influenced in any way by the patient's social situation (Böhme 1991).

*Other special issues*

The provision of care to relieve the pain and suffering of terminal patients is the joint duty of both medical doctors and nursing staff. If either neglect their obligations in this respect, this can be judged as negligence as specified in Criminal Code § 323c or as causing bodily injury through an act of omission according to Criminal Code § 323 in conjunction with § 13 (Federal Supreme Court, Böhme 1991).

Indirect active euthanasia for reasons of pain relief is exempt from punishment if the emphasis is on the relief of pain. In this case, the life-shortening side-effect of pain relief is accepted. Passive euthanasia, i. e. allowing the patient to die without his or her consent is exempt from punishment if the treatment is discontinued in the sense of a presumed consent after an unfavourable prognosis has been made. For the same reason, it is justified to turn off technical instruments and controls after an unfavourable prognosis.

Direct active euthanasia through killing is always a punishable offence. Even if the patient explicitly asks for euthanasia as a means of pain relief, it remains punishable (Criminal Code § 216, killing on request).

Summary of the relevant laws is included in Table 3.

**Table 3**. Summary of main laws related to autonomy, privacy and informed consent in Germany

| Concepts | Laws |
|---|---|
| **AUTONOMY** | |
| Personal liberty | The Constitution |
| | Criminal code |
| Self-determination | The Constitution |
| | Law of Social Care |
| Choice of hospital | Social Security Code |
| Insight into the files | |
| **INFORMED CONSENT** | Criminal code §226 |
| **PRIVACY** | |
| Protection of private secrets | Criminal code §202 |
| Privacy of the post | Criminal code §202 |
| (secrecy of correspondence) | |
| Confidentiality in legal action | Code of Criminal Procedure §52 |
| | Civil procedure §383 |
| | The "new" law of guardianship of 1994 |
| | Penal law |
| Presumed consent | § 677 German civil code |
| Avoidance of a suicide | Judgement of the Federal Supreme Court of 1984 |
| | Killing on request § 216 Criminal code |
| | Denial of assistance § 323 Criminal code |
| Social security institutions have the right | |
| to information | § 203 II No. 2 Criminal code |
| | § 1543 German National Insurance Code |

## 2.3 Greece

The examination of the legal issues that govern the doctor-patient relationship in Greek Law is of special theoretical and practical interest, not only because Greek literature and Law do not offer detailed solutions to the issues of the day, but also because the similarity of the Greek Civil Law to other European Laws, except for the Anglo-Saxon Law, justifies identical solutions to specific legal problems (Androulaki-Dimitriadi 1993).

The doctor-patient relationship is clearly a personal relationship, and this is also evident in the Civil Law. The nature of this relationship results in specific rules that are implemented in medical practice: these rules include confidentiality, informed consent and the freedom to choose one's attending physician. Nurses' relationship with patients come under the same rules. The nurses' responsibility for their services parallels medical responsibility but is autonomous (Anapliotou-Vazaiou 1993).

In Greece, human rights are protected by International Declarations and conventions on which the legal status of patients is based. The Greek Constitution of 1975 (Manessis & Papadimitriou 1986) refers to the right to health, saying that the state is responsible for the health of its citizens, especially for the protection of young people, the elderly and handicapped persons (Article 21, paragraph 3). It is in response to this constitutional provision that the new National Health System was recently introduced, charging it with the responsibility to protect the life and health of its citizens and to provide health services to all, equally and regardless of economic, social and professional status. In 1978, the Ministry of Health launched an effort to sensitise health professionals, especially physicians, to questions of bio-ethics, but it is only during the past ten years or so that there has been increasing interest in and public awareness of issues related to patient's rights.

Although patients' rights have been addressed in a number of different laws, it was in 1992 that legislation directly addressed the hospitalised patient's rights (Law No 2071, on Health System Reform, Article 47, 1992). Eight paragraphs in Article 47 of this Law deal with the rights of the hospitalised patient; the rights of prisoners are also protected by moral codes. Article 51 of the same Law establishes a National Board of Ethics and Deontology within the Ministry of Health, as well as local ethics committees in hospitals. The main purposes of the board are to set up a policy on ethical issues and to provide consultation.

*Autonomy*

The theory of autonomy constitutes the base for the principle of informed consent. Autonomy is the ability to think and decide, and to act according to that thinking and the decision. Autonomous persons are not only capable of expressing themselves freely, but they can also make choices and plans freely and base their actions on these plans (Anapliotou-Vazaiou 1993). The Greek philosopher Papanoutsos (1984) defined autonomy as another word for freedom, in its two meanings: freedom from causality and freedom in relation to ethical law that one can have formulated oneself or that can have been formulated by others. A somewhat different definition is given by a nurse, according to whom autonomy "is a form of personal freedom that relies on one's respect for human dignity. People have the right to determine the course of their life as far as there is no restriction to the autonomy of others. A person is considered as autonomous when he/she is capable of logical reasoning and self-guidance (Plati 1997).

According to Law 2071/92, Article 47, on the Rights of the Hospitalised Patient, the patient has the right to seek appropriate hospital services for his/her health problem (paragraph 1). The patient has the right to allow or refuse every diagnostic or therapeutic treatment. In cases of partial or complete mental incapability, this right can be protected by an authorised person (paragraph 3). Information given to the patient must allow the patient to form a complete picture of the medical, social and financial variables that must be considered in his/her condition; the patient must receive sufficient information to either to make informed decisions about himself/herself or to participate in decision-making which will influence his/her future life (paragraph 4). The Law states that the patient's collaboration, for research or educational purposes, can only be enlisted if the patient feels absolutely free in making the decision to collaborate or to refuse his/her collaboration. This consent can be withdrawn at any time (paragraph 5). The patient has the right to have his/her religious and ideological beliefs respected (paragraph 7). He/she has the right to make a complaint and to be fully informed about any progress in the matter as well as about the results (paragraph 8).

One of the fundamental principles in Greek medical services is the right of the patient to freely choose his or her physician. Although this principle derives from the general principle of respect of the patient's personality, it nonetheless remains quite theoretical and is indeed often tested by the practice of medicine today.

However, this right is secured from two perspectives. First, it is secured in negative terms in that the doctor cannot deny his or her services in an emergency situation: in Greek law this is recorded in the Penal Code (1985, Art. 307 and 441), the Greek Code of Medical Deontology (Art. 13) and the Code on the Practice of Medicine, enacted in 1939 (A.N. 1565, Article 25). Second, the law that established the National Health System in Greece in 1983 (E.S.Y.), even though it divides the country into health sectors, expressively gives patients the right freely to choose their doctor, even outside of their own health sector. In practice this is not always feasible as patients would have to travel long distances to obtain the services of the doctor of their choice, but the right nonetheless is there. This is particulary important in view of the character of the physician-patient relationship and the inherent limitations of the informed consent requirement.

*Privacy and confidentiality*

The right of the patient to demand that all information obtained or discovered by the doctor or nurse in the course of consultations, examinations and treatments shall remain confidential, is probably one of the oldest patient's rights.

The Greek Code of Medical Deontology (Politis 1990) recognizes the doctors' obligation to keep all medical information confidential irrespective of the scheme under which they are offering their services, i.e. whether they are working in the public or private sector (Article 18). Article 23 of the Code on the Practice of Medicine (1939) also refers to this patient right, providing that any breach of confidentiality is only legal when imposed by law.

The Penal Code (1985, Art. 371) states that members of the clergy, lawyers, doctors, nurses, midwives, pharmacists and their assistants who disclose confidential information that they have obtained in the course of or because of their professions or capacity, will be liable to a fine or imprisonment. The Penal Code thus seeks to protect the privacy of the patient in an effort to promote the public health. Moreover, the said code regulates the testimony that medical doctors may give in courts of law in view of the confidential information they possess.

The Civil Code (1984, Art. 57) recognizes and protects from any unlawful attack the individual's right to personality. The Greek Supreme Court's decision S.C. 60/1969 provides a precedent (Supreme Court Decision 1969).

The Penal Code does not offer any definition of the exact meaning of the term 'confidential information'. An event or information is regarded as confidential if it is known to a limited number of persons whose interest or wish dictates that this remains known by them and them alone.

However, the Penal Code states that the disclosure of confidential (medical) information is not unlawful when this is done to fulfil a duty, for example to declare a death, birth or infectious disease when required by law or to protect a right recognized by law or an essential interest that could not be protected otherwise. The existence of an essential interest cannot be determined by a general rule, but is judged on a case-to-case basis.

It is not clear in the Greek literature whether the doctor, nurse, midwife and their assistants can lawfully disclose confidential medical information with the patient's consent. There are advocates of both views.

The data protection is mentioned in Civil and Criminal Code and a more recent Law No 2472/1997 "Person's protection from personal data processing". This law institutes the requirements for personal data processing for protection of the rights and the ultimate freedom of persons, especially their private lives. In seven articles are reported all the information regarding

- The characteristics of personal data
- The conditions of data processing
- The information of the authority about the development of records and initiation of data processing
- The process of sensitive data
- The connection of records
- The personal data flow between countries (outside Europe)
- The confidentiality and safety of data processing

In six articles are reported information related to a function of authority concerning the protection of personal data. In three articles are reported the administrative and criminal penalties and the civil responsibility.

Moreover, it should be noticed that the principles of European Medical Deontology (Standing Committee of Doctors of the European Community 1987) are ingrained in Greek medical practice. Regarding confidentiality, Article 4 states that the doctor is the person most trusted by the patient and must therefore safeguard the confidentiality of all information obtained during their relationship. Medical confidentiality continues to apply after the patient's death. The doctor must respect the patient's private life and take all necessary precautions to ensure that no information obtained in the practice of his/her profession will be disclosed (Anapliotou-Vazaiou 1993). As far as the protection of electronic medical data is concerned, there is nothing in the Greek Law to prevent abuse; the only statement referring to the issue is in Article 8 of European Medical Deontology, stating that doctors cannot co-operate in the development of a medical data bank, as this would endanger or restrict the patient's rights to confidentiality, safety and the protection of his or her private life.

The Law of the Reform and Organization of Health System (No 2071/92, Article 47), makes it clear that the patient has the right to medical and nursing care that fully respects human dignity (paragraph 2). Every patient has the right to protection of his/her private life. The confidential nature of all patient information and documents, medical notes and findings relating to the patient must be guaranteed.

*Informed consent*

Medical paternalism finds justification in the Hippocratic Oath in which there is no direct reference to the patient's informed consent as a deontological principle. The concept of informed consent in medical care is a rather new medicolegal issue. The Hippocratic doctor demanded obedience from the patient; according to the Hippocratic Principle, a doctor-patient relationship was based on the doctor's good behaviour towards the patient (Anapliotou-Vazaiou 1993). The term 'consent' is defined by Koutselinis & Michalodimitrakis (1984) as the assent which the patient gives for the performance of all the medical interventions judged as necessary by the doctor. According to the encyclopaedia dictionary of Eleftheroudakis (1965), consent means agreement given of one's own free will; compliance; permission given for an action; mutual decision.

Closely related to the patient's free choice of doctor is the right of the patient to receive adequate information about the diagnosis, prognosis and available treatment(s) in order to make an informed decision on the course of the treatment that should be followed. Since every medical act entails some degree of intrusion, it is always required that the patient gives his or her informed consent, whether explicitly (oral or written) or implicitly.

Article 8 of the Code of Medical Deontology refers directly to informed consent, underlining the obligation of the medical doctor to respect the patient's personality and free will. In general informed consent, as viewed by international and Greek jurisprudence, should be serious and spontaneous, that is, it should correspond to the true wish of the patient and not be the product of deceit, pressure (psychological or physical) or blackmail. It should also be an informed decision. Greek courts have specified that the doctor should disclose the nature of the medical act that is proposed, alternative(s) to the latter, the consequences that are certainly known to follow (if there are such), potential risks and the foreseeable results. The doctor is not obliged to disclose *all* possible risks, but only those that a reasonable practitioner would disclose and a reasonable patient would need to know to make an informed decision.

As regards informed consent, the European Medical Deontology, Article 4 states that "Except in emergency situations, the doctor ought to inform the patient of the expected results and consequences of the treatment, in order to get his/her consent, especially when the suggested actions involve major risks" (Anapliotou-Vazaiou 1993). Greek Law supports the view that the obligation to provide information, which makes it illegal to attempt arbitrary medical practice, results from specific statements which concern specific cases but which can be considered as general principles. Such statements include e.g. Article 31, paragraph 2, and Article 33, paragraph 1, of the Morals Code. According to this Code, "every type of appropriate medical examination or medical surgery performed on a prisoner is allowed with the prisoner's consent" (Frantzeskaki 1990, 116). Doctors' responsibility to inform patients is regulated by the Civil Code, Articles 334 and 922.

According to Androulaki-Dimitriadi (1993), informing the patient is a medical duty. The person who informs the patient has to be a doctor. Delegating the informing of a patient to paramedical personnel or other non-doctors constitutes medical negligence. There are two sides to this matter:

▪ The non-medical personnel (including nurses) has no obligation to inform the patient, nor does the patient have the right to be informed by non-medical personnel; the physician and the hospital correspondingly have no right to delegate the informing of the patient to non-medical personnel.

- In a case where the patient has been correctly informed by non-medical personnel, the patient is considered informed and there is no medical negligence as the information essentially flows from the physician. The physician does have the obligation to be assured that the patient has been correctly informed. This view, indirectly, accepts the patient's receiving information from non-medical personnel. If the patient is informed, and informed correctly, the source of the information becomes inconsequential. The physician has to prove that the patient is informed. Androulaki-Dimitriadi (1993) also states that the para-medical or nursing personnel of an out-patient clinic, laboratory, hospital, health centre, or the like, has its own obligation to inform the patient about nursing activities (injections, minor operations, trauma care, physiotherapy etc.) that are part of the diagnostic and therapeutic treatment but performed under the responsibility of the para-medical personnel, since they are considered simple nursing activities of the daily medical practice. This again brings up the question of therapeutic information. In cases like these, and because the para-medical or nursing personnel acts under the supervision of the physician or, in some cases, of the hospital, the responsibility for negligence in informing the patient is attributable to the person performing the care as well as to the physician or the hospital.

The hospitalised patient's right to informed consent is included in Law 2071/92, Article 47. In the third paragraph, it is mentioned that the patient has the right to consent to or refuse any diagnostic or therapeutic practice that would be performed on him/her. In the case of a patient suffering from partial or total mental incompetence, this right is claimed by the patient's legal representative. The fourth and fifth paragraphs are also concerned with the patient's right to ask for information relating to his/her health condition in order to form a complete picture of the medical, social and financial parameters involved and to either make decisions for himself/herself or participate in decision-making which can affect his/her future life (paragraph 4). The patient has the right to be informed in advance about the possible risks involved in the implementation of unusual or experimental diagnostic and therapeutic measures. These measures can be implemented only after the patient's consent. This consent can be withdrawn at any time. The patient must feel free to refuse - or to agree - to collaborate in activities for research or educational purposes.

At this point it is useful to note that Greek law also specifies (albeit indirectly) the person that should give substitute consent in the case of a minor patient or a mentally ill patient. The persons that the Civil Code recognizes as the representatives of a minor and mentally ill person, or the persons mentioned in the Penal Code (1950, Art. 13), are those to whom the doctor should turn in those cases.

In the event of an emergency the doctor or nurse should act in the patient's best interests, regardless of whether they have obtained the latter's consent. They should act as sound practice would dictate in similar circumstances; otherwise they could be accused and prosecuted for omitting to save a person at risk (Penal Code 1985, Art. 307).

In the most recent Law No 2472 (1997) the subjects' rights on personal data processing are mentioned in four articles: the right to information (the responsible person has the obligation to inform the subjects and the authority for the data collection and processing), the right of access, objection, and temporal judicial protection.

*Special provisions*

Special provisions are made for certain patient categories, such as minors and prison inmates.

As has been pointed out earlier there are several legislative documents which refer to minors with respect to informed consent. However, unlike other European countries, Greece has no provisions to accept an age limit for informed consent lower than that of maturity. This certainly constitutes a shortcoming in Greek law.

Law 1329/83 introduced some changes to our Civil Code and among other things added a new article (1534) which gives the physician the right to act contrary to the will of the patient's parents or legal representative. This article was enacted primarily with a view to cases where Jehovah's Witnesses refuse to have a blood transfusion, but it applies to other situations as well.

It is also worth mentioning Article 102 paragraph 7 of the Code of the House of Correction (A.N. 125/1969), which states that interventions on the body of an imprisoned person are allowed only if his or her bodily integrity and life are in serious danger because of his or her refusal to receive food or because of a contagious disease. In such cases the prisoner can be forced or, in the latter case, be provided the appropriate vaccinations and treatment.

As far as euthanasia is concerned we should note that Greece has no special legislative documents pertaining to this important issue. Euthanasia is forbidden and is viewed by Greek law as murder. Article 300 of the Penal Code refers to the killing of a person upon serious and persistent demands. In this case the law says that the person letting or helping the patient die will be sentenced to imprisonment, but in contrast to the case of intentional murder this does not carry the death penalty or imprisonment for life. The situation is entirely different, however, if in the case of active or passive euthanasia the patient has not asked for help to die.

A final issue that deserves our attention here is that of experimentation. Apart from certain general clauses in the Code of Deontology and the Code on the practice of medicine, there are no important legislative provisions. Although there exist certain bodies that control the different protocols, their job is not very well defined in law. This is particularly noteworthy and unfortunate as quite a considerable number of studies are carried out in Greece each year.

*Conclusion*

Although there have been some efforts to create legislation in support of patients' rights in Greece, very little work is going on at the present time. This is a major problem that calls for the attention of strong interest groups. The protection and advancement of patients' rights will not only promote and enhance public health, but also strengthen the relationship between doctors and patients.

The foundation of Greek Medical Ethics and Deontology Association and the Ministry of Health have started to inform health professionals on matters related to medical ethics and patients' rights.


*2.4 Spain*

With the introduction of democracy in 1975, Spain has undergone important transformations. Various democratic projects emerged in the society to shape the new Spanish State. In 1978, the New Constitution was ratified by the new Spanish Courts. It was hoped that this would facilitate a process of agreement by consensus among the different projects, which would eventually form the bases of democracy. According to Abel (1990):" the three figures who sealed the pact were: first, the social democratic state by law that leaves the door open to establish and advance democratic society or total democracy, second, an autonomous state which joins the political unity of the state with a right to self-government of the nationalities and regions and finally, a non-denominational state that establishes the secularization of the state, while at the same time permitting religious freedom for both the people and communities."

In 1975, a new ethical mood which was characterized by a new language, the language of rights, new codes, patients rights and a new concept 'Bioethics' began to have many international repercussions. Spanish society, very sensitive to democratic values, rapidly incorporated in its new health laws all the changes that were happening in the field of medical Bioethics in the USA and Europe.

The new Spanish Constitution of 1978, focusing on the dignity of the human person, defends liberty, justice, equality and political diversity of ideologies as superior values and recognizes the following rights:

- To respect for life and physical and moral integrity (art. 15)
- To ideological and religious freedom (art 16.1)
- To liberty and security (art.17.1)
- To privacy (art. 18)
- To freely communicate and receive information (art.20)
- To participate in public matters(art. 23.1)
- To preserve health (art. 43)

This allows the principles of autonomy privacy and informed consent to be incorporated in the laws without breaching the constitution. The Spanish State should also follow the guidelines of the document of the Parliamentary Assembly of the Board of Europe (January 1996) drawn up by the Commission for Health and Social Affairs. The 18 members are invited to take pertinent measures in order to ensure that patients' rights are respected.

The process followed by Spain is very different from that of the USA. The judicial jurisprudence has not played the same role as in the Anglo-Saxon world. The judicial function in continental Europe is reduced almost exclusively to the application and interpretation of laws (Gracia 1989).

The legal formulation process of patients' rights has had unfortunate foundations. The Royal Decree 2082, 28th of August 1978, that contained a list of the patients rights in the state hospitals ("Seguro Obligatorio de Enfermedad") was considered invalid by the Supreme Court. Later, in October 1984, The National Health Institute set up a plan to make the health service more humane. Its basic aim was the development and articulation of a Bill of Rights and Obligations of the Patient. Its efficiency was practically zero. However the same letter was modified, and is actually included in the General Health Act (1986) In this way, the patients rights, have been given priority (Gracia 1989).

From this point onwards the Spanish Health Service has chosen a model of approach supportive of patient autonomy, in place of the old paternalistic model. However, due to the lack of tradition in this approach, some basic rights such as the right to die with dignity, or the right to religious assistance were forgotten (Gracia 1989). Catalonia was an exception here. Catalonia has managed to incorporate rights such as these into the Bill of Patients Rights of the Departament de Sanitat i Seguretat Social (1984) and this Bill of the Patients Rights is also included in the Hospitals' Accreditation Order (1991).

*Autonomy*

With the appearance of the Bill of Patients' Rights, the principle of autonomy acquired, for the first time, a precise formulation in terms of rights, despite this term not appearing explicitly in judicial terminology. The concept is nonetheless implicit in the majority of decrees.

The principle of autonomy is specified in the General Health Act of 1986 in art 10, parts 2,4,6,7 where the right of the patient to be informed of the health services, diagnostic procedures and therapies, are recognized. The patient should have a free choice among the different options presented by the doctor. Patients also have the right to refuse treatment. Part 5 affirms that the patients and his relatives have the right " to be given, in comprehensible terms, complete and continuous information, both verbal and in writing, concerning the process, including the diagnosis, prognosis, and alternative forms of treatment". It must be emphasized here that the idea that the family be informed at the same time as the patient could be said to be peculiar to the Latin culture; where the family has a great influence in comparison to that in Anglo-Saxon countries.

Decree 284/1996, regulated the Catalan System of Social Services. Although autonomy is not mentioned, essential rights necessary to facilitate the exercise autonomy are recognized. In Art. 5, Part A, the right to information is recognized, as is the right of patients to participate democratically in decisions which affect them. The right to relevant information is recognized as a necessary step in order for a person to be able to be autonomous. In Art. 7, access to Nursing Homes is regulated. It specifies that a person must previously have expressed his will and consent to being admitted to this type of care facility. In the case of an incompetent patient his legal representatives, or the judge, will determine whether the person shall be admitted or not.

The Civil Code in title IX, referring to incapacity states, in article 211, that "in the case of mental illness rendering a person incapable of deciding or consenting for himself, this person cannot be admitted for treatment without judicial action; except in cases of emergency, in which case it will be taken before a judge within 24 hours."

*Privacy*

The regulation of the right to privacy is recent in Spanish legislation and it is difficult to define according to that legislation. Spanish Law did not use the term "privacy" until recently, using "intimacy" in its place. Anglo-Saxon influence has changed this and notions of privacy appear in most recent laws. Now, one can find a great variety of terminologies, such as "intimacy", "private life", "private space" and "privacy" (Corbella 1996).

These terms are used in distinct ways, they refer to different areas of the human activity. The sphere of the individual is divided into three: the private area, which is made up of behavior, information or utterances that the subject wishes to keep from public knowledge. The confidential area includes the issues that the person shares with people in this trust. The secret area includes, knowledge events. etc ,that the person makes inaccessible to others and it is within this area that the term privacy is developed.

Corbella (1996) defines it as: "The right of each person to separate and keep to himself particular matters or aspects of his personality, as well as ideas, attitudes or individual behavior, which become part of the private life of the individual in virtue of a decision freely made, in brief, the right to not communicate it to the other people."

Spanish Laws which deal with issues relating to privacy are:

- The Spanish Constitution (1978)

In article 18; the fundamental right to intimacy is recognized specifying in the third point that intimacy includes safeguarding as secret one's utterances, in particular by telephone, by post, and by telegraph which may only be made known by judicial order. Individuals and public authorities both must respect this.

- Civil Code
- Organic Act 1/1982 of 5 May, on the civil protection of the right of honour, personal and family intimacy, highlights the fundamental right to intimacy and stresses that this is an essential and inalienable right.
- Organic Act 5/1992 of 29 October regulates the automatic treatment of data of a personal nature (LORTRAD). Regulates the protection of intimacy (confidentiality) of computerized data.
- Penal Code

The new Penal Code of 23-11-95, which came into effect on 24-5-96, gives penal protection to intimate (confidential) material. The articles 197-201 describe and sanction those crimes that affect intimacy (confidentiality); from the act of discovering or knowing without authorization, whatever a person keeps as secret until this is revealed.

- The General Health Act

The General Health Act of 25-4-86 in art. 10.3 affirms that everyone has a right " to confidentiality of all information related to the process and stay in private and public health institutions." Under the general law of health, the concept of confidentiality is understood as a shared secret. Confidentiality, which is not revealing any data, implies that a significant bond of trust be established between health workers and the patient.

Other laws within the health area also include confidentiality or intimacy in their articles. These are:

- Act of 35/1988 of 22 November that regulates the techniques of assisted human reproduction whereby it is explained that any information concerning the donor will be kept in the strictest confidentiality. Here, the concept of secret in place of confidentiality has been used in order to emphasize the idea of non-revelation.

- Act of 30/1979 of 27 October, and The Royal Decree 426/1980 of 22 February, which regulates the extraction and transplant of organs. This states that the identity of the receiver of the organ will be withheld.
- Decree 284/1996 of 23 July, of the regulation of the Catalan System of Social Services. This decree regulates assistance and social services, explicates the conditions for its operation, the characteristics of the services and social establishments. Included in this is a description of the rights of the users of long stay residences (Nursing Homes). In the article 5, part b, the right to intimacy and non-revelation of personal data which is found in the clinical records of the patients, are recognized.

*Informed consent*

With the Spanish Constitution of 1978 came the beginning of a new era in the history of Spain. It meant that finally paternalism had been overcome and a new model of social organization had come about, based on the idea that it is the sum total of the wills of each individual which makes a particular form of government legitimate. The European Community calls this model a "Social State of Right". Historically the emergence of a new political power would have to be followed by reforms in health service, meaning that the concept of autonomy would become known in different levels of society and finally reach the most private areas. (Simón 1996).

The right to informed consent is covered in the General Health Act. (1986) art. 10 part 4. The idea of informed consent in its first years had little support from the administrative bodies who had upheld it, (the "INSALUD", National Institution of Health. Ministry of Health). After 1993, increased public awareness stimulated and gave weight to its application in health care contexts, by demanding written consent forms. Doctors are now very sensitive to this, but their main concern is focused on the potential for litigation rather than respect for the right to autonomy of the patient.

In the research field, the earliest legislation is The Royal Decree 944/1978 of the 14 April that regulated clinical testing of pharmaceutical products and preparations. This brought about the setting up of clinical testing committees, predecessors of the actual Ethical Committee of Research. The Royal Decree did not specify the necessity for informed consent of those who participated in research, but only recommended that people should give their authorization. In 1982, the order that developed and extended this decree required that informed consent be obtained. Act, 25/1990 of 20 December (Medicine's Law), again updated this legislation and emphasized the necessity of informed consent. More recently the Royal Decree 561/1993 dedicates the entire art 12 to informed consent; an exhaustive review is given to the requirements of informed consent. This brings Spanish legislation into line with international declarations.

## 2.5 The United Kingdom

In the United Kingdom the awareness of patients' rights increased rapidly at the beginning of the 1990s. The official tone is set by the 'rights' and standards proclaimed in The Patient's Charter and by the recent organizational reforms to the National Health Service (NHS). The National Patients' Charter has had a major impact on public awareness of the performance of health care providers. It was introduced in 1991, and launched in 1991 as a management tool for improving standards. It is described as part of an overall trend to improve the quality of health services and give more value to the views of patients and carers. (WHO 1996a.)

The Patients' Charter outlined ten 'rights' and nine national standards. As an effect of this 'charterism', several care providers have adopted local charters with various kinds of principles, originating from the national charter. Yet the legal right of the individual to health care service, enforceable in court, is not emphasized in the United Kingdom. In general, the objective is to set a minimum standard throughout the country with local improvements. The idea of The Patient's Charter is to improve the quality of services and give more value to the views of patients and carers. Every citizen has the right to be registered with a general practitioner, and citizens may also change their doctor. Doctors may also choose their patients. However, patients have no rights to choose their specialist. (WHO 1996a.)

However, in considering the United Kingdom it needs to be remembered that within this unity there are four separate national units. "For many purposes the United Kingdom may be described as a unitary state, since there is no structure of federalism... (However) constitutional and legal differences exist within the United Kingdom and ... diversity, as well as political and economic unity, is found. While the legislative competence of Parliament extends to all the United Kingdom, three distinct legal systems exist, each with its own courts and legal profession, namely (a) England and Wales (b) Scotland (c) Northern Ireland. A unifying influence is that the House of Lords is the final court of appeal from all three jurisdictions, except for criminal cases in Scotland. When Parliament legislates, it may legislate for the whole United Kingdom (for example income tax or immigration), for Great Britain (for example, social security or trade union law) or separately for one or more of the countries within the United Kingdom." (Bradley & Ewing 1997, 45-46.)

Scotland, England (plus Wales) and Northern Ireland have entirely separate legal systems. They have entirely different roots. Since the Act of Union in 1703 the Scottish legal system is influenced by the English legal system. However Scotland has its own legal history, traditions, vocabulary and procedures. These are substantially different from those of England. Thus you have English and Scottish versions of relevant laws. There are some English laws for which there is no Scottish equivalent and vice-versa.

With in the context of this research project the UK representative is based in Scotland and data collection is restricted to Scotland. "Within the territorial limits designated Scotland the state has developed an organisation of courts and legal practitioners, a body of principles, rules and precepts, and a body of knowledge and thinking about law which amounts to the Scottish legal system. It is largely indigenous having grown and developed naturally within the country rather than being imposed from without, yet it is not narrowly parochial, having shared in drawing something from the legal systems of antiquity, nor yet insular, having a strong historical connections and logical affinities with legal systems of and derived from continental Europe. ... it is firmly rooted in general principles, so that much can be explained as deduction from, or detailed working out of, great overriding principles based on reason and justice." (Walker 1997, 23.)

In the UK based system many medico-legal matters which reach court and require a court decision are based on case law. However, there are a number of acts of parliament which are of relevance particularly in the area of patient autonomy and consent. The following are those identified as most pertinent.

*Privacy and confidentiality*

Issues concerning patients' privacy is included in the UK's law. Mason & McCall Smith (1994) suggest that the common law has long recognised the principle that every person has the right to have his bodily integrity protected against invasion by others. In medical treatment, every touching of the patient is potentially a battery (assault in Scotland) on that patient.

The Data Protection Act 1984 recognises the rights of individuals to personal information stored in computer banks. There is also a recognition in this area of legislation of the medical prerogative to prevent access to information which is "likely to cause serious harm". The latter is undefined. (Mason & McCall Smith 1994.) Access to Health Records Act 1990 (came into force in 1991) extends patients rights of access to health records prepared manually and held by a variety of health professionals. Patients have the right to see these records and the right to demand that any inaccuracies in the recorded information be corrected. Again, there is the possibility of withholding access to records likely to cause significant physical or mental harm. Rights of access do not apply to records made before 1991 (November). The Data Protection Act 1984 has now been replaced by the Data Protection Act 1998. The 1998 Act was a response to the EU Data Directive of 1995, and covers not only computerised data but also data which is manually stored e.g. in filing cabinets. In other respects the new Act is broadly similar to the 1984 Act.

*Informed consent*

Patients' consent has a strong meaning in UK law. As a general rule, medical treatment, even of a minor nature, should not proceed unless the doctor has first obtained the patient's consent. This consent may be expressed or implied, as it is when the patient presents himself to the doctor for examination and acquiesces in the suggested routine. This principle applies in the overwhelming majority of cases but there are limited circumstances in which a doctor may be entitled to proceed without this consent. Essentially, these can be subsumed under the heading of non-voluntary therapy which has to be distinguished from involuntary treatment. (Mason & McCall Smith 1994, 219.) Every citizen has the right to receive a clear explanation of any treatment proposed, including risks and alternatives, before the patients decide whether he or she will agree to the treatment. Citizens shall be given detailed information on local health services, including quality standards and maximum waiting times. (WHO 1996a.)

In the UK for valid consent to be obtained, the doctor must give the patient sufficient information to enable them to understand the nature and consequences of the proposed treatment. The courts recognize that a doctor may decide what is in the patients best interest to know, provided any decision to withhold information was reasonably made (Buchanan 1995).

According to The Patient's Charter (1991), the patient, if he/she wants, is entitled to accurate, relevant and understandable explanations of what is wrong with them; what the implications of this are; what can be done; what the treatment is likely to involve, and the patient is also entitled to a second opinion. The person who is carrying out the treatment should obtain consent for the treatment. However, if nurses are carrying out treatment which would usually be carried out by a doctor, the patient must be informed that the nurse isn't a doctor, he/she has just expanded his/her role (Friend 1996). This has to be done, in order to maintain the validity of the consent given. It is essential for a patient to be aware of the risks involved in a treatment in order to give fully informed consent (Tingle & Cribb 1995).

If not fully informed, and some risks occur, then the person can sue for negligence (eg. Sidaway v Board of Governors of the Bethlem Royal Hospital and the Maudsley Hospital 1984). In this case, a woman was left severely paralysed by an operation, and claimed that she wouldn't have agreed to the operation if she had been informed of all the risks. However, this is difficult to determine. A subjective test is used by the courts to decide whether the patient would still have agreed to the treatment had he/she had been given information of all the risks involved in the treatment (Chatterton v Gerson 1981). The patient left paralysed by the treatment sued for negligence, but lost the case, as it was stated that the neurosurgeon involved hadn't acted negligently. The Bolam Test (Bolam v Friern Hospital Management Committee 1957) is used to determine if there is a case of negligence. This test states that so long as a doctor has acted in accordance to the practice accepted as proper by a responsible body of medical practitioners, he isn't guilty of negligence.

In Britain, the law surrounding consent involves the doctor deciding how much information the patient should receive prior to consent being obtained, based on the above criteria (Tingle & Cribb 1995). There is no duty imposed on the doctor to point out every risk to a patient (Koergaonkar 1992); a doctor may decide what is in the patient's best interests to know, providing that any decision to withhold information was reasonably made. However, withholding information can deny the patient's right to autonomy and may increase anxiety (Buchanan 1995). This differs from the law in the USA, where the standards of disclosure of information is based on what the "prudent patient" would want to know. Although English law surrounding consent isn't likely to reach the American standard, in the near future, the amount of information a patient receives about his/her treatment is increasing.

Doctors usually provide patients with information, in order to obtain consent. However, factors within the doctor-patient relationship interfere with patient autonomy. For example, Besch (1979) found that patients trusted the recommendations of the doctor, and complied with them, without realising that a choice was being asked of them. Doctors can also make patients feel inhibited, and unable to express their fears to them, due to the social inequalities between them, and so are likely to comply with the doctors recommendations (Buchanan 1995). Involving a nurse in the doctor-patient consultation can be beneficial in some aspects of the consent process, as the nurse may be able to clarify what the doctor said, and answer any questions the patients may have (Kennett 1986), giving the patient time to make a decision.

Where the doctor is trying to obtain consent to treatment or surgery, the patient will be anxious, and anxiety is a barrier to communication. Thus, the patient may not be able to take in all that is said to him/her. Indeed, it has been found that in consultations, a lot of information is lost, through either a lack of understanding, or forgetting on the part of the patient (Ley 1982). Another factor affecting the obtaining of consent to treatments is that the place where the doctor is trying to obtain consent may affect patient understanding, eg. an unfamiliar hospital ward will make a person anxious, and so unlikely to retain all information.

Doctors often obtain consent in hospital wards, where there is a lack of privacy, and other patients can hear the consultation, through the thin hospital curtain. This lack of privacy may make the patient feel helpless, and unable to assert themselves enough to make a decision. Doctors must realise that although they think they know what is best for the patient in medical terms (Weiss 1985), it is the nurse who is in regular contact with the patient, and doctors obtain important information about the patient via the nurse. So, it would be beneficial to involve nurses more in medical decisions regarding patients.

In UK, a mentally competent adult has the right to refuse treatment. The Court of Appeal highlighted the importance of ensuring that when a patient refuses treatment, he/she has the mental capacity to make a valid decision, and hasn't been subjected to the undue influences of another person (eg Re T 1992, Dimond 1995). In such a case, where an individual has refused treatment on the basis of an outside influence, an authorising order may be sought, to allow the person to be treated. However, under the Mental Health Act (1983), patients who are seen to be incompetent to give consent, may be treated without consent being given. If the patient is not a legally competent adult, health care decisions can be made by the patient's parents, legal guardian, or, in some states, next of kin or friend.

The Principle of Necessity is normally used in arguments for non-voluntary treatment. Mason and McCall Smith (1994) comment that it is widely recognised in both criminal and civil law that there are certain circumstances in which acting out of necessity legitimates an otherwise wrongful act. The basis of this doctrine is that acting unlawfully is justified if the resulting good effect materially outweighs the consequences of adhering strictly to the law. In the present context, the doctor is justified, and should not have criminal or civil liability imposed upon him if the value which he seeks to protect is of greater weight than the wrongful act he performs - that is, treating without consent.

Necessity will be a viable defence to any proceedings for non-consensual treatment when an unconscious patient is involved and there is no known objection to treatment. The treatment undertaken, however, must not be more extensive than is required by the exigencies of the situation. (Mason & McCall Smith 1994, 220) - this position has now been extended to incompetent or incapax individuals in the case Re F (1989).

The issues of proxy consent has been discussed in the UK laws. Next of kin have no legal right to consent for an adult patient. Proxy consent is only truly valid if the person has given expressed authority to another person to give or withhold consent - or when the laws invests the person with such power - e.g. the parent child situation. In Scotland the Court of Session may appoint a tutor-dative who is then empowered with control of the personal welfare matters of an incapax (incompetent individual). Included in this is the power to consent to medical treatment on behalf of an incapax. This latter must be based on the best interests of the patient. Mason and McCall Smith (1994, 222) suggest that a doctor administering treatment to a child against parental wishes could rely on common law for support.

> "... the current judicial climate is such that we believe a decision taken in good faith in the best interests of the child would, save in very unusual circumstances, be upheld by the courts."

More detailed information concerning minors' rights is included in The Family Law Reform Act 1969. It gives minors between ages 16-18 the same rights of consent as an adult. Further, The Age of Legal capacity (Scotland) Act 1991 allows a minor who can demonstrate sufficient intelligent understanding of the issues to have treatment provided on the consent of the minor alone - although the attempt to obtain parental consent should be made nonetheless. In Scotland this supersedes the Family law Reform Act cited above - on the issue of consent. The issue of refusal of treatment is a lot less clear. It is not covered in this provision. However, The Children's Act in 1989 allows medical advisors to initiate proceedings against parents who refuse life saving treatment on religious or other grounds.

Legal guidance for the treatment of people with mental illness in the UK is found in the Mental Health Act 1983, the Mental Health (Scotland) Act 1984, and the Mental Health (Patients in the Community) Act 1995. The 1983 and 1984 Acts introduced major reforms in the treatment and review of involuntary patients and also considered issues of consent to certain forms of treatment In England the 1983 Act established a Mental Health Commission along the lines of the Scottish Mental Welfare Commission which had been established in 1960 (Mental Health (Scotland) Act 1960). Both of these bodies monitor admission procedures to hospitals and the conditions under which patients are detained. The 1995 act is primarily concerned with the after care of patients who have been hospitalised.

### 3. Professional codes in health care in Finland, Germany, Greece, Spain, and the United Kingdom

*3.1 General*

Professional ethics are important to the implementation of patients' rights (Nikkilä 1998). A professional code is an articulated statement of the role morality of the members of a profession (see Beauchamp & Childress 1994). A profession's standards can be seen at the micro-level, i.e. in how individual members behave towards their patients, clients and colleagues, or at the macro-level, where the professional ethic can be seen as something that the whole profession upholds and that can be invoked by individual members to support their behaviour. (Thompson et al. 1994.) The need for ethical guidelines has increased because, as Singleton and Dever (1991) have stated, today's complex, technologic and mechanical critical care settings present a large number of choices to the patient.

Professional codes are an important part of ethics. Professional groups which enjoy a monopoly in determining the service they provide must also accept responsibility for their standards of practice. From the profession's point of view, codes of ethics or codes of conduct are important as a means of giving their members some guidance as to their practice. (Thompson et al. 1994.) Codes do not state the obvious, and they are not law, but they do point to what should be (Tschudin 1986, Arndt 1996a).

Perhaps the oldest of the codes of ethics known, 'The Hippocratic Oath,' stresses all of the current issues of the importance of teaching and learning, the good of the patients and the avoidance of harm, the problems of abortion, the need to know one's limitations, professional conduct and confidentiality. (Downie & Calman 1994.) The content of the Hippocratic Oath is as follows:

> *I swear by Apollo the physician, by Aesculapius Hygeia and Panacea, and I take to witness all the gods all the goddesses to keep according to my ability and my judgement the following Oath. To consider dear to me as my parents him who taught me this art to live in common with him and if necessary to share my goods with him; to look upon his children as my own brothers to teach them this art if they so desire without fee or written promise to impart to my sons and the sons of the master who taught me and the disciples who have enrolled themselves and have agreed to the rules of the profession but to these alone, the precepts and the instruction I will prescribe regimen for the good of my patients according to my ability and my judgement and never do harm to anyone. To please no one will I prescribe a deadly drug, nor give advice which may cause his death. Nor will I give a woman a pessary to procure abortion. But I will preserve the purity of my life and my art I will not cut for stone, even for patients in whom the disease is manifest I will leave this operation to be performed by practitioners (specialists in this art). In every house where I come I will enter only for the good of my patients keeping myself far from all intentional ill doing and all seduction and especially from the pleasures of love with women or with men, be they free or slaves. All that may come to my knowledge in the exercise of my profession or outside of my profession or in daily commerce with men which ought not to be spread abroad, I will keep secret and will never reveal If I keep this oath faithfully, may I enjoy my life and practise my art respected by all men and in all times; but if I swerve from it or violate it may the reverse be my lot'*

In medicine, The World Medical Association has approved the Declaration of Lisbon (1981), the content of which was revised in 1995. This declaration reaffirms the patients' right to high quality medical services, self-determination, information and confidentiality, as well as their right to make informed choices. (Nikkilä 1998.)

The oldest norm that provides ethical guidelines for the nursing profession is the Florence Nightingale Pledge, dating from 1893. The Nightingale pledge has been adopted by many professional nursing organisations and groups. It has been written by

Canadian-born Lystra Gretter. This pledge reflects Florence Nightingale's philosophy and style (Deloughery 1995, 23):

> *I solemnly pledge myself before God, and in the presence of this assembly, to pass my life in purity and to practice my professional faithfully. I will abstain from whatever is deleterious and mischievous, and will not take or knowingly administer any harmful drug. I will do all in my power to maintain and elevate the standard of my profession, and will hold in confidence all personal matters committed to my keeping and all family affairs coming to my knowledge in the practice of my profession. With loyalty I will endeavor to aid the physician in his work, and devote myself to the welfare of those committed to my care.*

The first ethical rules for professional nurses were adopted by the American Nurses Association in 1953, and the International Code for Nurses was adopted in 1953 (ICN 1953, 1976, see also Johnstone 1989). The first ICN Code described the fundamental responsibility of nurses as threefold: 'to conserve life, to alleviate suffering and to promote health' (Tschudin 1986). The rules also specify four sets of duties for nurses: their duties to patients, to other nursing professionals, to co-workers, and to the organisation and society. At this point in time, ICN ethical codes have been published in almost all countries. The countries may also have special norms for research ethics in nursing science.

Another international code is the International Code of Ethics for Midwives, ICM (1993). The aim of the ICM is to improve the standard of care provided to women, babies and families throughout the world. This improvement comes from the development, education and appropriate practice of the professional midwife.

Furthermore, laboratory technologists have their own code, the Code of Ethics of the International Association of Medical Laboratory Technologists (IAMLT 1992). It is in ten parts, including the demand to maintain strict confidentiality of patient information and results and to safeguard the dignity and privacy of patients.

In the next few chapters, we will describe professional codes in Finland, Germany, Greece, Spain, and the United Kingdom.

*3.2 Finland*

In Finland, there are ethical codes for many professions; most of the codes have been revised in the 1980s and 1990s, and new ones are under preparation (Hannikainen 1992). These codes are rather similar in content, but they differ in emphasis (e.g. Kalkas & Sarvimäki 1994).

Nursing codes in Finland are based on ICN Codes (1973). Ethical Guidelines of Nursing have been approved by the Assembly of the Finnish Federation of Nurses in September 28, 1996. The aim of the ethical guidelines is to support nurses, midwives and public nurses in their everyday decision-making involving ethical questions (Tehy 1997). The guidelines are an expression of the basic aim of nurses and the ethical principles of their work, not only for the nurses themselves but also for other health care professionals and the general population.

The Ethical Guidelines are divided into six areas which discuss the mission of nurses, the relationship of nurses and patients, the work and professional competence of nurses, nurses and their colleagues, nurses and society, and nurses and their nursing profession. The nurse aims to support and increase the personal resources of individuals and improve their quality of life. The nurse is responsible for his/her actions, first and foremost, to the patients in need of help and care. The nurse protects human life and improves the individual well-being of the patient. He/she also encounters the patient as a valuable human being and creates a nursing environment which takes into consideration the values, convictions and traditions of individuals. (Tehy 1997.)

The nurse respects the autonomy and self-determination of the patient and gives him/her an opportunity to participate in decision-making about his/her own care. Nurses also realise that all the information given by the patient is confidential and judgement must be used in sharing this information with other people involved in nursing. The nurse treats the patient as a fellow human being; he/she listens to the patient and empathises with him/her. The relationship between nurse and patient is based upon open interaction and mutual trust. Furthermore, the nurse exercises impartiality in his/her work. He/she treats every patient equally well, according to the individual needs of the patient and irrespective of the illness, sex, age, creed, language, traditions, race, colour, political opinion or social status of the patient. And lastly, nurses have a responsibility to see that no professional involved in care acts unethically toward patients. (Tehy 1997.)

In Finland, the Ethical Guidelines of Nursing also support the midwife's everyday practice (Tehy 1997). Besides these Guidelines, Finnish midwives follow the International Code of Ethics for Midwives (ICM). The international code is in four parts: midwifery relationships, the practice of midwifery, the professional responsibilities, and the advancement of midwifery knowledge in practice. (International Confederation of Midwives 1993.)

The Finnish Union of Practical Nurses called Super (Suomen lähi- ja perushoitajaliitto 1996) has also drafted ethical guidelines for practical nurses. The profession of practical nurse is still relatively new in Finland; it takes the place of earlier school-level vocational qualifications in social and health care. Super concentrates on the values and principles of care and the caring professions. The four principles are as follows: respect for human dignity, self-determination, equality and justice. The principle of self-determination is based on the belief that each person is the best expert on his/her own life. For customers or patients to be able to make decisions about their own treatment and care, they need to be given sufficient information about different services, alternative methods of treatment and their effects. The ethical guidelines make it clear that an autonomous person is capable of independent reflection and decision-making. The person also has the right to follow the course of action determined by his/her reflections and to receive appropriate assistance. (The Finnish Union of Practical Nurses 1996.)

The different professional groups in health care have their own ethical codes in Finland: radiographers (Suomen Röntgenhoitajaliitto 1992), practical children's nurses (Suomen Lastenhoitoalan liitto 1993), practical mental nurses (Finnish Federation of Mental Health Nurses (Suomen mielenterveyshoitajaliitto 1997), physiotherapists (Suomen fysioterapeuttien eettiset periaatteet 1998), the Finnish Association of Intensive Care (Suomen Tehohoitoyhdistys, STHY 1997) and laboratory technologists, who follow the Code of Ethics of the International Association of Medical Laboratory Technologists (IAMLT 1992).

The Finnish Medical Association adopted its first ethical guidelines in 1956. They were based on the Declarations of Geneva and the International Code of Medical Ethics. Additions were made to the guidelines in 1963, and in 1988 the Association adopted revised ethical guidelines and a code of collegiality. (Lääkärin etiikka 1996.) There are eleven items in these guidelines.

*3.3 Germany*

How are the three concepts understood in German nursing? This question cannot be answered by a translated enumeration from a German code for nursing ethics. It is necessary to present a brief account of the historical background relevant to the development of ethical codes in post-war Germany.

When after 1948 the human rights movement with its declarative manifestations took hold, professional bodies in all wakes of services formulated or reformulated their own specific ethos. This was to demonstrate the at-oneness of any given profession with the ideals of the human rights movement. Especially in the area of health care services this was to be a definitive commitment to respecting the human dignity of clients, their autonomy, their rights and their freedom from coercion. Thus, the medical and legal professions for instance issued statements and statutory rules as to their professional and moral integrity.

Likewise the German nursing community found itself at the beginning of forming a new identity after the shattering experiences of the Third Reich. As from 1945 the *Controlling Council* representing the allies (Britain, France, America, and Russia) was responsible for legislation regarding commerce and trade, the constitution or reconstitution of political parties, and of specific professional or otherwise oriented organisations. One of the statutes of the *Controlling Council* forbade the constitution of any centrally administered and organised nation-wide association, union, or federation. This accounts for the strengthening of small local interest groups trying to promulgate nursing's plight. Thus, the different churches and denominations, the church-dependant bodies and charities, the religious orders, the Trade Unions, the local Red Cross associations, and various other independent charities founded their own local nursing associations.

In 1954, when with the Treaty of Paris German sovereignty was reinstituted many associations, federations, and groupings aspired to national status, and endeavoured national unity of their hitherto locally dispersed subgroups. This accounts for the fact that German nursing is represented in a many-faceted fashion. Unlike in other countries there is no national professional body in Germany which represents all nurses and which is responsible for professional practice. Federal legislation and the criminal law safeguard good practice in nursing and in midwifery. The membership in the above mentioned organisations is comparatively small; a rough estimate is that about 7-10% of German nurses and midwives are members of professional organisations.

However, already in 1954 the ICN Code of Ethics was translated by the German professional nurses union (DBfK), the largest independent association. It was widely circulated and generally used in nurse education in West Germany. In order to demonstrate their professional concern and their political and moral accountability most of the various associations formulated some ethical guidelines within the frameworks of their statutes. Such statements emphasised priorities of religious or political underpinnings of ethical issues in nursing.

In 1985 new federal legislation made the teaching of ethics to nursing students compulsory. With a renewed interest in ethics during the last ten years most associations and federations produced new and more articulate ethical guidelines relating to various fields of practice. During the course of this the DBfK translated the ICN publication by Sarah Fry into German (Fry 1995). This book emphasises the concepts of autonomy, informed consent and privacy based on the 1973 reformulated ICN Code of Ethics for Nurses.

In the former German Democratic Republic (GDR) the Socialist Union Party (SED) assumed responsibility for the cultural, professional and the moral education in all areas. No specific ethical codes for nurses or midwives were in existance, but the official curricula stated some political and moral baselines applicable to practice (Ministerium für Gesundheitswesen 1985). Introductory sentences pointed to the need to ground all professional knowledge in Marxist-Leninist teachings. A socialistic-humanist professional ethos was to further personal development in learning and working. The unity of politics and morality was said to be the presupposition for the realisation of the health care politics of the SED (Ministerium für Gesundheitswesen 1985).

In East Germany Catholic Orders were allowed to maintain their existance if they applied themselves to healthcare or the social services. Thus, communication on various matters of Church teachings penetrated via the West German branches of those orders to the East. Also a branch of the Catholic Caritas Nurses Federation was in existance, thus contacts were used to exchange knowledge and news. Especially during the 1980s undercover seminars were held by West German members of the Caritas Nurses Federation in various Dioceses in East Germany. Disguised as visitors catholic nurse teachers thus made ethics texts on nursing known in the East. For this purpose a translation of the Irish Guild of Catholic Nurses Code was used (Caritas Gemeinschaft 1987). Further, retired catholic lay nurses as well as religious who had permission to visit the West smuggeled ethics material through the Iron Curtain.

Similarly Protestant Nurses Federations, and Deaconesses held inofficial contacts. Especially the Berlin branches were active insupplying their East Berlin colleagues with information and material related to professional and ethical issues.

After Unification in 1990 the West German nurses associations and federations be they independant or associated with the Churches opened local branches in the East. Especially the DBfK developed strong activities here.

In an attempt to provide an overview of the current state of emphasis on the concepts of autonomy, privacy, and informed consent in German nursing Codes and Statutes, they will be addressed as they feature in the various texts of the main associations and federations. The following documents form the basis of this synopsis:

- Anonymous (1995) Wittenberger Thesen - Vorschläge zum ersten Kontakt mit der Psychiatrie
- Arbeitsgemeinschaft katholischer Pflegeorganisationen (1995) Die ethische Verantwortung der Pflegeberufe

- Caritas Gemeinschaft für Pflege und Sozialberufe e.V; Deutscher Caritas Verband e.V., and Katholischer Berufsverband für Pflegeberufe e.V. (1998)
- Caritas Schwesternschaft e.V. (1987) Ethik im Pflegealltag. Zwangslage der Moral für Krankenschwestern und -pfleger in einer sich verändernden Gesellschaft. (Irish Guid of Catholic Nurses: Moral Dilemmas for Nurses in a changing society
- Behindertenhilfe (1995) Ethische Grundaussagen der vier Fachverbände der Behindertenhilfe
- Deutscher Berufsverband für Pflegeberufe e.V. (1992) Berufsordnung des DBfK.
- Deutscher Berufsverband für Pflegeberufe e.V. (1995) Die Herausforderung Gesundheit 2000 - Implikationen für die Pflegeberufe
- Evangelischer Fachverband für Kranken und Sozialpflege (1993/94) Ethische Leitlinien.
- Martens, E. (1995) Ethik-Kodex, Ethische Grundregeln der Altenpflege
- Schwesternschaft des Ev. Diakonievereins e.V. (1996) Pflege- und Dienstverständnis der Schwestern im Ev. Diakonieverein
- Strunk, H. (1995) Ethische Regeln der Intensivpflegenden (Ethik-Kodex)
- Verband der Schwesternschaften vom Deutschen Roten Kreuz (1995) Berufsethische Grundsätze der Schwesternschaften vom Deutschen Roten Kreuz

*Autonomy*

Some texts link the specific perspective of nursing specialities to the ICN Code and present very general points (Martens 1995, Strunk 1995). Most codes or statutes recourse to the declaration of human rights and derive the concept of autonomy from there. Thus, the fulfilment, maintenance, and safeguarding of basic human rights feature prominently in the fundamental ethics statements of the associations for the assistance and care for handicapped people (Behindertenhilfe 1995).

The DBfK document (Deutscher Berufsverband für Pflegeberufe e.V. 1992) states that each person has a right to professional nursing care and must be protected from untoward practice, and that respect for the dignity and value of human life is part of nursing. Nurses will foster the autonomy of clients and their families in all phases of their life.

German Red Cross nurses maintain that their perception of good nursing includes the respect for patient's autonomy and the right of patients to freely make their own decisions regarding treatment and care (Verband der Schwesternschaften vom Deutschen Roten Kreuz 1995).

Catholic nurses derive their concept of patients' autonomy from a view of human sovereignty being a divine gift and thus commanding the nurses' respect for the autonomy of patients. In a joint publication of catholic organisations involved in health care services it is stated that each person is to be viewed as a subject, which needs to be given the greatest possible amount of autonomy (Arbeitsgemeinschaft katholischer Pflegeorganisationen 1995, Caritas Gemeinschaft für Pflege und Sozialberufe 1998). Human existence is not chance happening but embedded in God's will. But herein all people have a high degree of freedom and self-determination which is to be upheld by health care workers. Autonomy is seen as a value, which can come to the fore, by the application of the nursing process (Caritas Gemeinschaft für Pflege und Sozialberufe 1998). The power of experts and the autonomy of patients are juxtaposed but should not be in conflict with each other. Questions of power, powerlessness, and helplessness must be addressed in order to find valid answers and mutually acceptable rules (Caritas Gemeinschaft für Pflege und Sozialberufe 1998). The workgroup of Catholic Nurses' Organisations emphasise that vulnerable patients are not to be left without assistance, help, and advise in difficult situations, here the principle of solidarity supplements the autonomy principle. Respect for the autonomy of patients can be demonstrated in the way and manner patients are addressed and their needs and wishes are elicited and heeded (Arbeitsgemeinschaft katholischer Pflegeorganisationen (1995).

The protestant stance focuses on the objectives of (nursing) being support and attention. Nurses ascertain the greatest possible independence and autonomy for the sick and for handicapped people. They promote a patient's inner growth and maturity, so that he may acknowledge his own personal path towards faith (Evangelischer Fachverband für Kranken und Sozialpflege (1993/94).

Intensive Care nurses acknowledge the right of their patients to independence, autonomy, and self-care (Strunk 1995).

*Privacy*

The concept of privacy is rarely addressed. It features indirectly in the protestant understanding of nursing as a service. It is alluded to in the context of caring for the dying, where dignity has to be preserved in all nursing circumstances and situations. This is underpinned by saying that every person is created by God and made to attain union with God. This fact is the source of a person's dignity which is inviolable and thus to be protected (Schwesternschaft des Ev. Diakonievereins e.V. 1996).

In the ethics code for intensive care nurses the notion of privacy is directly addressed with the statement that intensive care nurses maintain and defend the right of patients to privacy, this includes the safeguarding of personal data (Strunk 1995). A similar sentence is found in the Irish Nurses Code where the right to privacy is emphasised and related to the careful handling of personal data (Caritas Schwesternschaft e.V. 1987).

In relation to people's first contacts with psychiatric institutions a set of Theses has been formulated by psychiatric nurses (Anonymous 1995). They state that respect for personal preferences regarding physical contact; nearness or distancing, communal life or privacy needs to be upheld. Personal responsibility (autonomy) should be fostered and strengthened, knowing that self-healing abilities are active in each psychotic episode. The choice of 'recovery spaces' in times of crisis should be made freely. Even in acute psychotic situations, personal preferences are to be heeded (Anonymous 1995).

*Informed consent*

The DBfK code of professional conduct emphasise the right of the individual, their significant others, and their family to obtain comprehensive information about their state of health in order to participate in decision-making (regarding their own health). It further states that nurses will inform the public about health matters (Deutscher Berufsverband für Pflegeberufe e.V. 1992). This socio-political perspective is taken up in a recent paper regarding the topic of Health 2000. The DBfK recommends that the public needs to be involved with discussions related to ethical questions concerning the social and health services (Deutscher Berufsverband für Pflegeberufe e.V. 1995).

This is further emphasised in the public debate in Germany about the European Bioethics Convention (see Bockenheimer-Lucius 1995, Rössler 1996).

The Red Cross nurses promulgate the need to secure patients free and uncoerced decisions regarding their treatment or non-treatment. This applies in the same manner to nurses' actions as it does to medical treatment (Verband der Schwesternschaften vom Deutschen Roten Kreuz 1995).

From the Catholic perspective respect for patients' autonomy calls for the right to informed consent. Patients must be included as far as possible in any decisions to be made (regarding their health) (Arbeitsgemeinschaft katholischer Pflegeorganisationen 1995). This is echoed by the protestant view that (Christian) nurses heed the right (of any person) to make their own decisions and to be independent (Schwesternschaft des Ev. Diakonievereins e.V. 1996). Further, patients are respected as persons and in their individuality, therefore a patient will be informed in a comprehensible manner as far as possible - taking heed of his condition – of any measure to be taken. Patients are partners in the process of decision –making, they have personal responsibilities which should be upheld and fostered (Evangelischer Fachverband für Kranken und Sozialpflege (1993/94).

The code for intensive care nurses states that patients in intensive care, because of the severity of their conditions often cannot express their needs, their fears and their concerns, intensive care nurses therefore act sensitively as advocates for their patients and the next of kin of their patients (Strunk 1995).

The Theses regarding ethical conduct towards psychiatric patients point out that information as to treatment and side-effects of treatment is to be given as soon as possible, above all information as to personal rights must not be withheld. Giving information is not a singular event, but must be ongoing and it must include patient's' relatives' (Anonymous 1995).

*3.4 Greece*

The debate on autonomy and self-determination versus the benefit of the patient has been going on since the birth of scientific medicine, and it continues even today. Doctors and nurses continuously confront events and conditions that force them to decide whether to put the principle of beneficence before the principle of autonomy. This remains a highly topical bio-ethical problem.

Hippocrates, the founder of scientific medicine, was interested in the nursing care of the patient. In his writings on the "Techniki" that nowadays we call nursing, patient care is described in detail (Mandilaras 1994). The care emphasis in medicine is close to that in nursing, and Hippocrates' suggestions for physicians' behaviour and morals can be considered to apply to nurses as well. The suggestions are found in his books, and the Hippocratic Oath for physicians is accepted throughout the world. This same oath is given by Greek nurses upon graduation.

The principle of nonmaleficence, one of the most important ethical principles, comes from the Hippocratic Oath which states that the physician shall protect the patient from any harm or injustice. The physician's primary obligation is to use all his/her knowledge for the benefit of the patient. In the era of Hippocrates, medical paternalism was based on the principle of beneficence, and it took the form of total obedience of the patient to the physician. The view that the benefit of the person has priority over his/her autonomy is evident in "Peri Eyschimocinis" by Hippocrates. In "Parangeliai," he even presents the physician as the only person responsible and capable of judging what is beneficial for the patient. The only right of the patient that Hippocrates recognises is the right of selecting the physician. However, after the selection of attending physician, the patient owes total obedience to his/her orders (Mandilaras 1994).

Plato's "Politeia" subscribes to the view that the patient can judge what is best for him/her; this may not always be the extension of his/her life. Plato also recognises the patient's right to change physicians or to refuse therapy. This view indicates real respect of the patient's autonomy and right for self-determination (Gryparis 1997).

The history of medical ethics dates back to the Hippocratic period. The Hippocratic Oath was the first Medical Code of Ethics, and today, 25 centuries later, all universal and professional oaths and codes are still based on it (Rigatos 1991a). Rigators (1991b) has listed all medical codes and declarations applied in medicine today. Specific situations such as clinical trials on drugs and HIV examinations in humans, are regulated by Ministerial Decisions No 10983 (1984) and Circular No 4548 (1990).

Nursing Code of Ethics (1996) in Greece is based on the International Code of Ethics of the ICN (1973), the Nursing Code of the American Nurses Association (1976), Codes of Nursing Ethics for the European Countries, the Declaration of Helsinki (1976), the European Map of the Rights of Patients' (1984) and the Principles of the European Medical Deontology (1987).

Nursing Code of Ethics (1996) consists of 27 Articles covering different topics, such as the general duties of nurses, relations between nurses, doctors and other health care professionals, and the duties of the nurses: research and collaboration with public services for the promotion of public health.

A major part of the code deals with the nurse's duty to the patient. To be more specific, Articles 5 and 9 make it clear that the nurse owes absolute respect to the patient's personality, sense of personal freedom and decisions. He/she must protect the rights of the patient and use all means necessary to prevent any kind of abuse. Articles 10 and 11 focus on information that the nurse gives to the patient about the diagnosis, the treatment, the prognosis, the risks and the requirement of the patient's informed consent before each nursing and medical intervention. At the same time, the nurse must respect the privacy of the patient. He/she must not do anything that can damage the confidentiality of patient data. Nursing interventions always presuppose the patients' ethical autonomy and freedom of choice.

*3.5 Spain*

*Nursing codes*

The first code of the Spanish State was written in 1985 by a group of nurses who felt the professional responsibility to respond to the political changes undergone in Spain and the necessities of a society, which was very sensitive to the problems of values and human rights. Twenty-two nurses took part in its preparation, representing the different specialties in nursing. During a period of two years, periodic meetings took place with 0the object of reaching complete agreement on the different criteria. This private initiative had the support of the "Institut Borja de Bioètica". One year later, in 1986, the professional nursing bodies of Catalonia democratically passed this same code. Know as "Ethical code of Nursing" which is still in force today. This code incorporates the values of the new Spanish democracy, which are listed in the new Spanish Constitution. It recognizes the autonomy of the patient (Arts, 6,7,8) and dedicates various articles to the need for information so that the person can be autonomous (Arts, 18,19,20,21.22). It emphasizes the right to privacy (Arts 23,24,25,26,27,28,29) without expressly mentioning informed consent.

Three years later, 1989, The National Board of Professional Colleges in Spain drew up the "Deontological code of the Spanish Nursing" with representatives from the different Professional Colleges of Spain. This code would be in force in all Spain except Catalonia. Given that many more people were involved in drawing this up, it was much more difficult to reach such precise conclusions. This difficulty is evident in the final version of the Code. This Code is much more general and less precise in the more conflictive aspects than that passed in Catalonia. At the time it was draw up, the new General Health Law had been passed, in which articles dealing with informed consent were incorporated (art. 7,8,9, 17) at the same time it deals with the topics of information (Art, 10,11,12,13) and intimacy or professional secret (Art 14,19,20,21).

*Guidelines*

Besides the different laws protecting autonomy, informed consent and privacy rights, the Ministerio de Sanidad and Consejerias de Sanidad (Ministeries)of different areas have elaborated guidelines in order to accomplish legislation. The following are some examples:

- Guia de Recomanacions sobre el Consentiment Informat (Guidelines of Informed Consent). Conselleria de Sanitat. Generalitat de Catalunya (Ministry of Health Catalonian Autonomous Government). This document emphasizes the importance of correct information, and it adopts the definition of Informed Consent definition used by the Royal College American Physicians. It highlights the importance of the nurse's role in the process of informed consent.
- Guia practica del Consentimiento Informado (Guidelines of Informed Consent) Comunidad Foral de Navarra (Autonomous Government of Navarra). This does not explain the role of the nurses.

- Pla de Salut de Catalunya (Catalonian Health Plan) In this document the Ministry of Health of Catalonia explains the health objectives for the next two years in Catalonia. The introduction of informed consent is one of these.

## 3.6 The United Kingdom

There are two key documents in the United Kingdom: Code of Professional Conduct for Nurses, Midwives and Health Visitors (UKCC 1992) and Guidelines for Professional Practice (UKCC 1996). The Code of Professional Conduct, revised in 1992, sets out clearly that the individual registered practitioner in the UK is personally and professionally responsible and accountable for all of his or her actions. The Code is composed of a stem sentence and 16 clauses. The first clause commands the nurse to "act always in such a manner as to promote and safeguard the interests and well being of patients and clients."

The UKCC Code of Professional Conduct (1992) states that each registered nurse, midwife and health visitor must always act in such a way to safeguard and promote the interests of individual patients and clients. They must also recognise and respect the uniqueness and dignity of each patient, and respect the need for care, irrespective of their ethnic origin; religious beliefs; personal attributes, the nature of their health problems, or any other factor. However, these guidelines suggest that the patient must be told the truth about his/her care, and be fully informed about risks involved in treatment, so that he/she can make the best decision.

In contradiction to this, the UKCC (1992) also supports clinical discretion, involving the right to withhold information from patients, which will prevent them making a fully informed decision, although it states that the decision to withhold information must be justified. These guidelines place the nurse in conflict between her duty to her patients, and her professional obligation to go may along with doctors decisions to withhold information from patients.

The other clauses in the Code of Professional Conduct give direction on the following:

- the involvement of patients and relatives in decisions regarding health care;
- the need to work in a collaborative manner with patients, relatives and other staff;
- the requirement that the nurse to recognise limits to his or her competence and knowledge;
- the requirement, on the professional to maintain and increase professional knowledge and competence;
- the need to respect the dignity and individuality of each patient
- what to do in a case of conscientious objection to a proposed line of treatment;
- avoiding misuse of the privileged relationship which the nurse has with a patient
- maintaining patient confidentiality;
- the nurse's responsibility to report to appropriate authority any thing in the care environment which may pose a threat to a patient;
- the nurse's responsibility when the health or safety of a colleague seems at risk;
- the nurse's responsibility in supervising or supporting less experienced colleagues or care workers in the development of their skills.
- receiving gifts or hospitality from patients.

- The prohibition against using one's registered status for advertising purposes.

In relation to notions of patient autonomy clause 1 requires the nurse always to act to promote the best interests of the patient. Clause 5 requires the nurse to work in an open an co-operative manner with the patient and relatives in order to promote the patient's independence and to recognise the right of the patient to be involved in decisions regarding his or her care. Clause 7 draws attention to the duty of the nurse to respect the uniqueness and dignity of the patient and clause 10 requires the nurse to protect the patient's confidentiality.

Following criticism of the Code from both within and outside the profession, and in the light of many inquiries to the UKCC seeking clarification on what the Code required of the nurse in particular circumstances, UKCC decided to develop more explicit guidance for the profession of what was being required of the individual practitioner by the Code of Professional Conduct.

There was wide consultation throughout the profession in the UK regarding what was required. The UKCC then produced a booklet called Guidelines for Professional Practice in 1996. This document explains the thinking behind the clauses in the Code and makes clearer that the Code cannot provide explicit detailed procedures to be followed in cases of ethical difficulty. It highlights the need for professional, moral judgement on the part of the individual practitioner, in the knowledge of the demands of the Code of Professional Practice and recognising the UK legislation relevant to the particular practice context.

For example, gaining consent from patients is often seen as the business of doctors rather than nurses. However, this has been disputed, due to the fact that the nurse is so involved with the patient (UKCC 1992). Thus, legally, the nurses should have a role to play in gaining consent. Most of the time, medical care involves obtaining written consent, and nurses often find themselves involved in such processes. The nurse could be found guilty of negligence, if the patient was harmed as a result of being given wrong or inadequate information.

At the end of the Guidelines a list of the documents and laws which are relevant to the Guidelines are provided. These are reproduced below.

Documents relevant to the Guidelines:
- Code of Professional Conduct, UKCC, 1992
- The Scope of Professional Practice, UKCC, 1992
- Midwives Rules, UKCC, 1993
- The Midwives Code of Practice, UKCC, 1994
- Standards for Records and Record Keeping, UKCC, 1993
- Standards for the Administration of Medicines, UKCC, 1992
- Confidentiality: use of computers, position statement, UKCC, 1992
- Complementary Therapies, position statement, UKCC, 1995
- Acquired Immune Deficiency Syndrome and Human Immune Deficiecy Virus Infection (AIDS and HIV infection), UKCC, 1994
- Anonymous Testing for the Prevalence of the Human Immune Deficiency Virus (HIV), UKCC, 1994.

These documents are available on request from the Distribution Department at the UKCC.

Laws relevant to the Guidelines
- Nurses, Midwives and Health Visitors Acts, 1979 and 1992
- Family Law Reform Act 1969
- Age of Legal Capacity (Scotland) Act 1991
- Children Act 1989
- Mental Health (Northern Ireland) Order 1986
- Mental health (England and Wales) Act 1983
- Mental Health (Scotland) Act 1984
- Abortion Act (1967)
- Human Fertilisation and Embryo Act 1990
- Data Protection Act 1984
- Access Modification Act(Health) Order 1987
- Computer Misuse Act 1990
- European Community Directive 91/507/EEC

Copies of these documents may be obtained from Her Majesty's Stationary Office (HMSO).

# Patient's autonomy in the literature

## 1. General

The modern medical era which started after World War II, might be called the Age of Autonomy (Siegler 1985). Nüremberg was a particularly important watershed in the annals of law and biomedical ethics, giving central importance to the principle of patient autonomy (Burt 1996). Thomasma (1983) has also described the post-war movement that has stressed personal development, individual ethical responsibility, and the importance of each gesture in day-to-day life, as opposed to community standards, political authority and social obligation.

In the late 1960s the citizens' right movement played a major role in strengthening individual rights to self-determination, focusing on such areas as education, working conditions and health and, within the health sector, biomedical research and prevention programmes (Riis 1987). Especially in the US ethical and legal analysis of medical decision-making has very much revolved around the idea of patient autonomy for the past 25 years (Blackhall et al. 1995). Autonomy is the guiding principle in US medicine and is highly valued because its exercise serves as a reaffirmation of the worth of each individual (Teres 1993).

However, the concept of autonomy has different meanings in different cultures. According to Gracia (1993), Mediterranean philosophers have been more influenced by European philosophy, particularly by Rationalism and Idealism, than by the Empiricist and Pragmatic Anglo-American tradition. In the concrete field of ethics, this means that the deontologic and principalistic approaches have predominated over teleological approaches and consequentialism. This explains why, for instance, the term "autonomy" acquired a different meaning in America than it did Europe. In US ethics, autonomy is defined as an "empirical" concept, as the capacity to act intentionally, with understanding and without controlling influences. On the contrary, European ethicists often interpret the principle of autonomy as a "transcendental" term in the Kantian sense, that is to say, as the capacity of human reason to impose absolute moral laws upon itself. In all Mediterranean countries respect for patient autonomy and patient rights to make decisions about their own bodies has grown considerably during the past few decades.

In the nursing literature, autonomy relates primarily to three areas: the discipline's desire for professional status, the impact of the socialisation of women and nurses, and the relationship of autonomy to job satisfaction within bureaucracies (Ballou 1998). In this chapter, however, our main focus is on patients' autonomy. A database search was carried out on Medline express using the keywords "autonomy" and "patient autonomy". Between 1965 and 1998, a total of 5657 abstracts have been published on different related subjects. The search with the keyword "patient autonomy" produced a total of 271 abstracts (see also Proot et al. 1998). Manual analysis of the abstracts and publications revealed a greater number of empirical studies in this field.

## 2. The concept of autonomy

The word "autonomy" is derived from the Greek autos ("self") and nomos ("rule", "governance", or "law"). It was first used to refer to the self-rule or self-governance of independent Hellenic city-states. Autonomy has since been extended to individuals and has acquired meanings as diverse as self-governance, liberty rights, privacy, individual choice, freedom of the will, causing one's behaviour and being one's own person (Beauchamp & Childress 1994). Autonomy can then refer to persons, their will, or an action in society (Gale 1989).

Autonomy has many champions. According to Thomasma (1983), Kant made the concept the heart of his moral theory by proposing that the self, through duty, is the ultimate origin of law. Similarly, John Stuart Mill proposed that a person cannot interfere in the freedom of others unless they may cause harm or cannot foresee the consequences of their action.

There are a number of problems relating to the concept of autonomy. Autonomy is very broadly defined (Gale 1989) and there is no consensus on a universal definition (Hertz 1996). Little agreement exists about its nature and strength or about specific rights connected with autonomy (Beauchamp & Childress 1994). Definitions proposed for purposes of direct observation have also proved problematic (Keenan 1999). According to Ballou (1998), the concept of autonomy is often confused with related concepts such as authority, accountability, power and independence. The concept is also difficult to articulate in practice (McCormack 1993). In addition, autonomy seems not to be a univocal concept, but several ideas constitute the concept (Horowitz et al. 1991). Further, problems occur when we talk about autonomy in everyday practice, although Castellucci (1998) has recently said that there are improved methods for defining and measuring autonomy that have contributed to the knowledge of the nursing profession.

## 3. Dimensions of the concept of autonomy

Autonomy can be defined from different perspectives (Table 4).

**Table 4.** Perspectives on the concept of autonomy

| Perspectives | Authors |
|---|---|
| Polarities | Collopy 1988 |
| Attributes | Hertz 1996 |
| Levels | Marieb 1992 |
| Approaches | Brazier 1987 |

Collopy (1988) identifies the following six polarities in autonomy:

- decisional autonomy versus autonomy of execution;
- direct versus delegated autonomy;
- competent versus incapacitated autonomy;
- authentic versus unauthentic autonomy;
- immediate versus long-range autonomy; and
- negative versus positive autonomy.

Further, Collopy et al. (1991) make a distinction between decisional autonomy (decision-making) and executional autonomy (implementing decisions). The risk for nursing practice is that decisional autonomy can easily be denied when executional autonomy is diminished or lost.

Hertz (1996) suggests the following defining attributes for autonomy: voluntariness, individuality and self-direction. Voluntariness implies the presence of choice, freedom from coercion, access to information and other resources, unrestrained thought or movement, and unconstrained decisions or behaviours. Both dependent and independent behaviours may be voluntarily chosen. Individuality includes having distinguishing characteristics, possessing a human uniqueness, being a distinct entity, and having a sense of self and knowledge of one's needs and goals. This denotes the idea that persons can recognise their own need for maintaining social bonds as well as their rights to privacy. Finally, there is the attribute of self-direction; subsumed within this attribute are guiding or controlling one's destiny, moving towards self-determined goals, and conducting one's own affairs. Self-direction may be exhibited by conducting one's own affairs to meet needs for both dependence and independence either separately or simultaneously.

A distinction can be made between three levels of autonomy. The first, physiological level, involves an autonomous process being characterised by its independence from other autonomous processes (e.g. Marieb 1992). The second, personal level, refers to the determining and defining self, which suggests a liberty to act in accordance with one's will, having independent thought and control over choice (Shotter 1975). The final level of autonomy is the social level. This highlights the fact that although social outcomes can be a direct result of an individual's intended actions, a model of autonomy must take constraining factors into account.

There are also different approaches to studying the realisation of autonomy (Brazier 1987). The first approach suggests that anyone over the age of an infant is autonomous, although autonomy can be lost with age (i.e. senility). The approach goes on to suggest that a person's view must be accepted, even in the absence of reason, thereby allowing the person to make mistakes. The second approach takes account of rationality and clear judgement in autonomy, and autonomy is considered to be a matter of degree, rather than all-or-none. It follows that the more rational and deliberate a person's actions are, the more choice they are allowed. The individual must show that they are doing the right things, for the right reasons, and there is little freedom to make mistakes. Both approaches outline different groups of people as autonomous. The first approach allows most people to be autonomous, while the second approach is likely to be a constraining factor on the autonomy of most people at some point, as no one can fully rationalise every decision they make (Brazier 1987).

The preconditions for autonomy are as follows: the integrity of the human body should never be violated; the curtailment of freedom should be in the interests of the people concerned; restrictions of liberty should also be for the furtherance of the common good (Dupuis 1987). Hertz (1996) uses the word indicators to describe the conditions for the presence of autonomy: the absence of physical, chemical or legal restraints on behaviours or decision-making indicates voluntariness; a person who refuses to follow the directives of others may exhibit voluntariness or individuality; this could be exhibited in dependent or independent behaviours; an individual uses the words which reflect individuality. Fourthly, a person who communicates desires and preferences exhibits individuality. Fifthly, by communicating goals, decisions, and rationale, self-direction is manifested. And lastly, following one's own plan whether to meet needs for dependence or independence is also evidence of self-direction.

According to Boladeras (1998), the principle of autonomy presupposes two ideas. First, a recognition of the fundamental value of individual free choice concerning life plans and the personal adaptation of ideals of human excellence. Second, the state and other individuals must not interfere in this choice or adoption. Dworkin (1988) has analysed autonomy as a concept that can rarely be found in a pure form: attaining autonomy depends on certain conditions. These are the ability to make independent choices; freedom from coercion; rational/reflective thought, and adequate information and knowledge. This suggests that the concept of autonomy is fragile, inconsistent and dependent on individual circumstances. However, despite the inconsistency of autonomy, Dworkin (1988) has identified two features that are common to all definitions of autonomy: that it relates to persons, and that it is a desirable attribute. A third feature is that all definitions contain, or should contain, the word "self", e.g. "self-rule", "self-determination", "self-government". Autonomy is based on the general recognition that an individual has unconditional worth with the capacity to determine his or her own destiny (Beauchamp & Childress 1994).

The concept of freedom seems to be included in autonomy. Papanoutsos (1984), for example, says that autonomy is another sense of freedom including two meanings: freedom towards the physical causality and freedom towards the ethical law which someone else has formulated (worded, outlined). For Plati (1997), autonomy is a form of personal freedom that relies on respect of human value. Persons have the right to determine the course of their life as far as there are no restrictions to the autonomy of others. A person is considered autonomous when he or she is capable of logical reasoning and self-guidance. Further, according to Thomasma (1984), autonomy includes the concept of 'freedom': the freedom from obstacles to carrying out one's desires; the freedom to know one's options; the freedom to choose goals, and to relate means to goals; the freedom to act; the freedom to create new options. However, the link between the concepts of autonomy and freedom is not clear (see Dworkin 1988, Scott 1998).

Autonomy has also been described from the perspective of decisions and actions. In practical terms, autonomy means that people have the right to make their own decisions, the only constraint being that their decisions should not interfere adversely with others, even if, by their decisions, they constitute a risk to themselves (Watson 1994). In addition, it means the persons have the right to determine their course of action on the basis of a plan which they have developed for themselves (Davies 1983). It includes the right to act freely, to make free choices, and to think as a person wishes

(Newman & Brown 1996). Further, Amelung (1992) includes participation in and control of medical decisions in autonomy.

Wright (1987) says that autonomous decisions are based on individual values and are made by utilising adequate information and understanding, free from coercion or restraint, and based on reason and deliberation. Horowitz et al. (1991, 23) suggest that autonomy is "the exercise of self-determined, goal-oriented behaviour that is or can be potentially threatened or inhibited by a variety of circumstances, real or symbolic, intrinsic or external to the person". Drawing on a concept analysis, Keenan (1999, 561) has provided an operational definition of autonomy, even though he was unable to find any way to directly observe autonomy: according to him autonomy is the "exercise of considered, independent judgement to effect a desirable outcome." Proot et al. (1998), for their part, conducted a concept analysis of autonomy in relation to the rehabilitation of stroke patients. Analysis of the literature showed that in the field of biomedical ethics, there are three central concepts of autonomy: self-governance, self-realisation and actual autonomy. In everyday nursing, autonomy means that individuals should be respected and their human rights upheld. This has a number of features, such as ensuring that people are not treated against their will, that they are informed about their treatment and about nursing care, and that they are involved in the decision-making process regarding that care (Johnstone 1989).

We may conclude that autonomy can be examined from different perspectives and that there are certain preconditions for its realisation so that decision-making is possible (Figure 2).

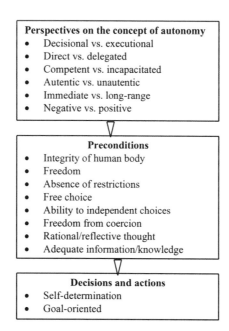

**Figure 2.** Dimensions of the concept of autonomy

## 4. Realisation of autonomy

The discussion below describes the autonomous person and factors supporting the individual person's autonomy.

### *4.1 Factors supporting autonomy*

Discussions on the various factors that can support autonomy (Figure 3) often focus on the individual's ability to make autonomous decisions or self-determined choices. Implicit in this is the notion of respect for people as rational, logical and important in themselves and not as mere means to the ends of others (McCormack 1993). Downie & Calman (1994) have observed that to be an autonomous person is to have the ability to be able to formulate and carry out one's own plans or policies. A second feature is the ability to govern one's conduct by rules or values. This suggests that to be autonomous means to be in control of one's life. This involves the individual being self-governing and self-ruled.

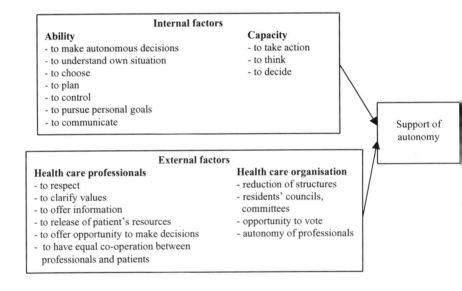

**Figure 3.** Factors supporting autonomy

Brown et al. (1992) have defined autonomy as consisting in self-determination, involving the ability to understand one's own situation, to deliberate, to make plans and choices and to pursue personal goals. The authors go on to propose that autonomy affirms the individual's sovereignty over his/her own life, so that if the individual's personal values conflict with those of another individual, that person has a responsibility to respect and facilitate the person's self-determination in making decisions. This suggests that autonomy involves not only the individual being self-determining, but also the individual respecting the self-determination of others. Gillon (1986) describes autonomy as the capacity to think, decide and act on the basis of such thought and decision freely and independently and without hindrance.

Autonomy rests fundamentally on the capacity to take action. It is defined as the capacity to think and decide independently (competence), the capacity to act on the basis of that decision, and the ability to communicate in some way with other people (British Medical Association 1995). An autonomous person is one who acts in accordance with a freely self-chosen and informed plan (Beauchamp & Childress 1994). When the will and liberty of decision-making is fully used, and when there is a certain balance between the will and decisions and liberties of others, we speak of an autonomous person (van der Arend & Gastmans 1996, Arndt 1996a,b, 1997, 1998b).

The aspect of capacity is also highlighted by Wright (1987) that persons are autonomous in the sense in which they are capable of formulating and acting on conceptions of how their lives should be lived. Autonomous agents can conceive of future alternatives. They understand they can pursue different ends and employ different means. In addition, autonomous persons can recognize conflicts between different ends and control their behavior in order to pursue those ends considered most valuable. Therefore, as Davies et al. (1997) have stated, there is a challenge for nursing practice to recognise when an individual is capable of making autonomous decisions.

In situations where a patient cannot function as his/her own autonomous, free agent, someone else must make the decisions which should be based on the person's beliefs and values (see Abades & Gasull 1995). The most obvious agent is the one designated by the patient (Marchette et al. 1993). Veach (1977) recommends that persons concerned about the quality of their terminal care designate someone who can support their autonomy and act in the person's best interest. Ideally, the designated person should have intimate knowledge of the functioning necessary for the patient to consider quality of life adequate. In the United States, "best interest" standards are used in deciding what medical care to provide to incompetent patients. This standard guides the incompetent's surrogate, whether family member, physician, court-appointed guardian, or some other decision-maker, to select those medical interventions that will most benefit the patient (Emanuel 1987).

There are various ways in which to support patient autonomy in the field of health care. However, the physician can have a position of obvious superiority with professional competence, while the patient is vulnerable and defenceless. Although autonomous as a person, the patient has to seek advice and help, seemingly from specialist (Camps 1999). On the other hand, doctors have the responsibility to maximise patient involvement in their treatment and to encourage and enable us to make fully informed, valid decisions about what happens to our own bodies (Bard 1990).

The nurse's role as patient advocate is an example of the way in which a nurse can help the patient, by defending his/her rights and helping him/her make autonomous decisions (Cahill 1994). The nurse can act as a mediator between the health professional and the patient, by explaining to the patient information inadequately explained by some other health professional. Some hospitals have employed persons, usually nurses, called patient relations coordinators, to respond to patient complaints and problems. The most effective hope for patient advocates, however, is in nurses intelligently involved in patient care. More than any other health professionals, nurses have frequent opportunities to facilitate and manifest respect for patients' rights (Bandman & Bandman 1995).

Health professionals can help to increase the autonomy of an individual by providing them with information on how to make their own decisions. The UKCC Guidelines for Professional Practice (1996) have been published for this purpose. Marchette et al. (1993) have observed that nurses should actively participate in decision-making that will foster the best interests of their patients. Nurses, as patient advocates, are usually aware of their patients' relevant values and beliefs and often find them to be in conflict with the medical treatment plan, causing ethical dilemmas.

How, then, can patient autonomy be promoted in practice? The notion of the patient having the right to participate in the decision-making process is one that can be fostered in patient-centred practice (McCormack 1993). Bailey (1994) says that helping the patient to maintain as much self-determination as possible will enhance mutual respect and trust in the doctor-patient relationship. This is more likely to be accomplished by providing information necessary for the patient to make informed decisions about what treatment plan, if any, will be followed. Collopy (1988) goes on to describe the support for the individual autonomy of dependent elderly people, suggesting that staff should recognise personal autonomy, even when a certain amount of decision-making must be delegated or when executional autonomy has to be substituted.

There are different ways in which patient autonomy can be supported (Arndt 1996a,b). First, by releasing, developing and focusing on the resources of the patients. Second, by offering patients the opportunity to make autonomous decisions. Third, by cooperation between nurses and patients in which the nurse has given up his or her dominating position. Therefore, we need to develop a philosophical, religious and moral model in nursing practice. Some other practical ways to foster self-determination and empower residents in nursing homes have been offered in an article by Lewis (1995), who refers to resident councils, different committees, resident newsletters, opportunity to vote, quality-of-life or dietary surveys, etc. Further, residents should be supported in the care planning process.

Illhardt (1985) describes two ways of supporting patient autonomy: first, by using self-help groups to help patients perform and cope with their life again; and second, by renunciation of patronising behaviour in the company of the dying. According to Juchli (1994), we should motivate patients to act more flexibly and try to reduce hierarchic structures.

In psychiatric settings, Altmann and Münch (1997) have described the concept of self-determination by psychiatric patients (n = 26). According to their results, self-determination, to psychiatric patients, means to carry through one's own wishes and ideas, to make decisions, and to coordinate and have influence on one's own affairs. They suggest that nurses can promote psychiatric patients' self-determination by giving them time, by asking patients' wishes, by supporting patients to act in a self-determined way, by giving information, by behaving in a polite manner, and by pointing out that self-determination is possible in restricted environments.

Spirig (1996) studied dying persons with AIDS (n = 8) using qualitative methods. The main areas relating to autonomy were control (being in one's own room), change, voluntariness and turning back. Spiring also discussed the question of how nurses could support patients' self-determination. She suggests, first, that nurses should develop and translate into action specific knowledge like concepts of control, changing, voluntariness, turning back and identification; second, that nurses should reflect on the understanding of caring from patients' point of view; and third, patients should have the right to use a single room and to lock the door. This would give the patient the opportunity to control his or her life.

Different tools and methods have been used in evaluating patients' competence levels; these include OARS (Older American Resources Scale), CIDDM (International Code for the Handicapped and Disabled) and MMSE (Mini Mental State Examination). These seem to be useful for measurements in the mental, physical and social spheres, but they are not adequate for analysis of the patient as a whole or patients' values. Yet these aspects are crucial in the situation where an elderly person no longer is in possession of all his or her faculties and is unable to make autonomous decisions but must rely on help from others (Abades & Gasull 1995).

Doukas & McCullough (1991) developed an instrument to enhance patient autonomy called the Values History. The instrument helps the health care team clarify the patients' expressed values when decision-making by the patient in no longer possible. The 'Values History' has two parts. The first section is an explicit identification of values, which invites the patient to identify those values and beliefs associated with terminal care that are most important to him or her. The second section is the articulation of advance directives based on the patients' values. This begins with acute care designations: consent for or refusal of cardiopulmonary resuscitation, use of a respirator and placement of an endotracheal tube. The chronic care designations then follow and include decisions for administering intravenous fluids, enteral feeding tubes, and total parenteral nutrition for nutrition support, use of medication and use of dialysis. However, it has been argued that health professionals should help the patient to be self-determining, even if this involves letting them make mistakes, and gain experience from this (Peckham 1997).

The autonomy of health professionals has also been discussed in connection with patient well-being. The Patient's Charter (1991) in the United Kingdom says that the autonomy of the patient can challenge the autonomy of the nurse, in relation to the patient complying with care. Porter (1992) states that the professional autonomy of nurses is at odds with the increasing trend towards patient empowerment. The drive now is to increase the autonomy of the patient, while nurses still have little autonomy. However, autonomous nursing can be enhanced by collaborative case management and primary nursing. Further, the balance of power between the nurse and the patient is influenced by the role adopted by the nurse (Morse 1991, Hewison 1995), as the traditional role of the nurse may disempower the patient by creating a parent-child relationship (Malin & Teasdale 1991). On the other hand, it has been pointed out that the role of the nurse facilitates the patient's choice, and empowers the patient (Wade 1995).

*4.2 Factors restricting autonomy*

There are many practical situations in everyday nursing where patients' autonomy may be restricted. These restrictions are based on the fact that autonomy is not an absolute right (see Aiken & Catalano 1994). The first limitation comes from the concern to minimise harm to the patient him- or herself. If it is in the best interest of the patient, then his or her autonomy can be limited or removed (Bard 1990). The second limitation comes from outside the person. We are not free to interfere in the rights, freedom and autonomy of other people (Bard 1990, British Medical Association 1995).

Factors restricting autonomy can be divided into two main groups (Figure 4), viz. internal and external factors (Veatch & Fry 1987). Internal constraining factors are all such that relate to the person him- or herself. These may be age, different forms of physical or moral dependency, ambitions, or individual circumstances.

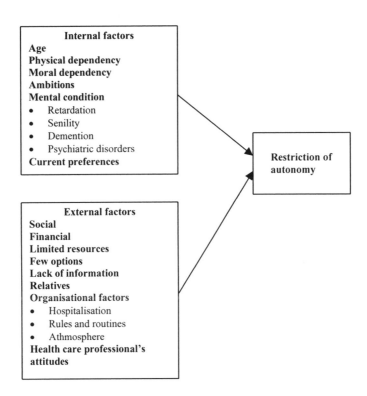

**Figure 4.** Factors restricting autonomy

One boundary to autonomy is the relationship of competence to behaviour and free choice. The principle of autonomy does not apply equally to persons who are immature, ignorant, or coerced (Newman & Brown 1996). Therefore, some individuals, because of their physical or mental condition, have diminished autonomy (Davies 1983). Examples are patients with mild mental retardation, young children and adolescents, those who become increasingly senile (Bandman & Bandman 1995), demented (Watson 1994) or persons with seriously psychiatric disorders (van der Arend & Gastmans 1996, Priami & Plati 1997, Välimäki 1998).

There may be times in mental illness, for instance, where autonomy is overridden and individuals can be treated forcibly for such illness against their will. Such procedures can be carried out if the mental condition is temporary and treatable and in situations where, in their normal mental state, individuals would not wish to constitute a danger to themselves or others (Watson 1994). In this case, the proxy decision-maker considers him/herself in the position of the individual in question and decides what the person would want if competent to decide. A person of diminished autonomy may be (partially) controlled by others or incapable of formulating or acting upon his or her own plans (Beauchamp & Childress 1994).

A distinction has been made between true autonomy and a person's current preferences. By yielding to a person's current preferences, a patient's autonomy is diminished rather than enhanced because refusing treatment due to an irrational fear, for instance, is not seen to be a reflection of true autonomy (Lindley 1991). Some people, although given autonomous choices, make non-autonomous choices, e.g. by signing a consent form without reading it (Beauchamp & Childress 1994). Further, although autonomy and respect for autonomy are highly significant, and are based on the idea that the individual can determine his or her own destiny (see Beachamp & Childress 1994), opposite situations may arise in practice. When the individual goes to hospital, he/she may assume the role of a passive recipient of health care (Abrams 1978). This passive role can be discussed in terms of the patient-professional relationship, where the patient is expected to be compliant and passive, while the professional takes on the role of guardian of knowledge and information, guiding the patient. It is through a lack of knowledge concerning his/her condition and treatment, as well as the frightening environment and intimidating health professional, that the patient may be too afraid to ask questions. It may then be assumed that the patient may either not want information, or may not be able to understand it (Byrne et al. 1988, Lavelle-Jones et al. 1993). This prevents the patient from being autonomous.

Further, some patients may not want to be autonomous. Biley (1992) published a small-scale study of patients' attitudes towards participating in decision-making, and found that the key responses to this were: "if I know enough" (knowledge); "if I am well enough" (strength), and "if I can" (organisational constraints). Thus, due to a combination of factors, some patients may not actually want to be autonomous regarding their care. They may believe that health professionals are better placed than them to make decisions regarding their care, and so pass the responsibility onto the health professionals.

External factors limiting patient autonomy may include financial position and social class (Seedhouse 1992). Brody (1980) highlights the problem of the "social gap", observing that physicians provide more information to those in higher social classes than lower social classes. Further, social tradition (Seedhouse 1992) or social interaction may also affect patient autonomy. For example, the elderly patient does not only suffer from physiological impairment but also in terms of disruption in personal and social interaction, which may not be due to ageing at all. Patients' autonomy may also be restricted by limited resources (British Medical Association 1995). Other important constraints on autonomy involve having very few options (Brody 1980), law (Seedhouse 1992, British Medical Association 1995) or relatives (Elander & Hermerén 1989).

Organisational factors are an important aspect of patient autonomy. That patients need advocates in the first place carries the assumption that there is a reduction in autonomy, and that patients' rights may not be respected (Willard 1996). Hospitalisation itself entails restrictions on patient autonomy and the exercise of preferences. This is due to rules and regulations which are interpreted and complied to in different ways depending on the situation and the people involved (Bergman & Goldander 1982). Because of their social situation institutionalised populations also tend to have less autonomy in their daily lives than the ordinary person (Davies 1983). Changes frequently associated with ageing, such as diminished vision and hearing, can contribute to lessened comprehension. Older clients may also experience great anxiety at the prospect of losing their independence as a result of the circumstances leading to hospitalisation or as a result of the effects of a chronic illness or injury on functional ability (McElmurry & Zabrocki 1989).

Elander & Hermerén (1989) found that organisational issues may present an obstacle to patient's autonomy. These may include the atmosphere in the hospital, hospital organisation, and rules and routines of the hospital (Elander et al. 1993). The attitudes of nursing staff decide to what extent patients are able to retain their autonomy. For example, the elderly are more inclined to relinquish their autonomy, since they were brought up when belief in authority was more pronounced than it is today. Patients in general are eager to behave themselves and to fit in with the hospital system; they are afraid of causing trouble and thus suppress their desire for self-determination (Elander et al. 1993). There appears to be strong evidence that physician values may play a more decisive role than patient values in many of these life-sustaining decisions (Orenlicher 1992).

Lack of information about one's own treatment may cause obstacles to the exercise of autonomy in an institution. Despite the value of giving information to patients and the promotion of joint decisions in patient care, there is a risk that nurses may withhold information from patients, thereby excluding them from decision-making and fostering a relationship of passivity and dependence (McCormack 1993). McElmurry and Zabrocki (1989) say that an important question here is whether autonomy is possible if an older patient has not received adequate information about his or her treatment and care, or does not understand completely what has been said. Perhaps rather more worrying in the face of possible threats to patient autonomy is the paternalistic tendency to assume either that patients do not want information, or that they would be unable to understand it if it were given (Byrne et al. 1988, Lavelle-Jones et al. 1993). Although patients are expected to take an active part in their care, it has been questioned whether patients actually welcome this role in nursing (Waterworth & Luker 1990, May 1995).

## 5. Autonomy in empirical studies

### 5.1 General

It has been argued that several studies on autonomy have been concerned with the question of paternalism in health care, its forms and influences (Delgado 1996). However, hardly any studies refer to maternalism.

Not every patient is necessarily interested in participating in his/her treatment and care. Ende et al. (1989) found that patients' preferences for decision-making in general were weak, while younger patients expressed stronger preferences. As patients were asked to consider increasingly severe illness, their desires to make decisions themselves declined. Patients who were less interested in making decisions themselves were more satisfied with how decisions were being made, and more satisfied with their medical care. However, there was no association between patients' decision-making scores and the number of times they had visited the clinic. In addition, there was no correlation between patients' desires for information and their preferences for decision-making. Those who preferred more decision-making in minor than in major illness, were better educated than those whose preference was strongest in major illness. In addition, they found that patients prefer the physician to take the major role as decision-maker, especially in severe illness. The most important positive correlate of a patient's preference for making decisions is younger age. Other variables associated with stronger preference for decision-making were higher education level, higher income, higher level of occupation, and divorced or separated marital status. Finally, patients who were more ill preferred lesser roles in decision-making.

There are certain cultural connections with the concept of autonomy, which can be identified in a study by Ip et al. (1998) who reviewed the literature on cross-cultural interactions in medicine between Western and Hong Kong traditions. Studies were selected that contrasted the approaches of different cultures to common ethical dilemmas in medicine. Review articles examining the relationship between culture and ethics were also selected. Hong Kong presents an interesting case study because of the coexistence of Western and Chinese medicine in a predominantly Chinese population that practises many Chinese cultural traditions. Whereas contemporary Western medical ethics focuses on individual rights, autonomy and self-determination, traditional Chinese societies place greater emphasis on such community values as harmony, responsibility and respect for parents and ancestors. Specific areas of cross-cultural conflict include: the role of the patient and family in medical decision-making; the disclosure of unfavourable medical information to critically ill patients; the discussion of advance directives or code status with patients; and the withholding or withdrawal of life support.

## 5.2 Autonomy and care of the elderly and chronically ill

The elderly population is growing in most Western countries. Most elderly people suffer from at least one or more chronic diseases, and they also have more contacts with physicians. The elderly are most typically treated in institutional settings, so maintaining client autonomy is the key issue in the moral treatment of the aged and chronically ill (Muyskens 1982).

An elderly person who is ill is nonetheless an autonomous person. Being hard of hearing, requiring time to answer, not being able to assimilate new information quickly, to mention only a few of the common factors found amongst the elderly, does not incapacitate them when making decisions concerning health care and their own lives (Barbero 1996). However, when adults become classified as elderly, there is a tendency for the principle of respect for autonomy to be rejected on the basis of incompetence and incapacity for decision-making (Chadwick & Tadd 1992). This view is supported by the fact that old persons often suffer a breakdown not only of physiological functioning, but also of social and personal interaction. They are also part and parcel of the psychosocial environment that encourages or discourages independence, participation in decision-making and personal worth (Bergman & Goldander 1982). Therefore, admission to a long-term care unit may in itself involve a drastic change in the terms of a person's existence, giving rise to strong feelings both in the patient and in his or her relatives, feelings of despair, aggressiveness, apathy and guilt (e.g. Elander et al. 1993).

A central issue in the care of the elderly is whether or not they can maintain a level of independence, and what risks they pose to themselves. There is the question of whether or not assertiveness to choose self-care and refuse help means they have a right to this, regardless of the risks involved. However, it has been stated that with the right to choice comes the responsibility of being accountable for one's actions, although the elderly with dementia, for instance, are not seen as accountable for their actions. It is stated that it is difficult to measure the extent of risk for an elderly person who is cognitively impaired and living independently. Despite impairments, it is important to give patients independence, even if it does carry risks (Watkins 1993).

A process of disempowering is often in evidence in the treatment of elderly patients. This was the case in a study by McWilliam et al. (1994), who collected their data in a document review and by means of observations and in-depth interviews. Informants included 21 patients, 22 informal caregivers, and 117 professionals. The study showed that lack of clarity about goals, aspirations and purpose in life and a general negative frame of mind in the elderly combine with professional practice approaches to create a disempowering process. Those patients with a positive mindset and sense of direction and purpose in life did not experience any threat to their autonomy. Therefore, it is important to enable elderly patients to maintain autonomy despite continued health care requirements.

Focus of empirical studies in autonomy of elderly patients are focused in six areas:

> ➤ Quality of care and attitudes of personnel to care
> ➤ Patients' wishes and needs
> ➤ Nursing activities
> ➤ Patients' nutrition and feeding
> ➤ Dressing
> ➤ Cultural issues

*Quality of care and the attitudes of personnel to care*

Issues of patient autonomy have also been discussed in studies relating to the quality of care. For example, Davies et al. (1997) reviewed empirical studies which have attempted to measure the quality of nursing care for older people in varied settings. They found some objective indicators to recur repeatedly. These included, firstly, implementation of systems of care delivery which promote comprehensive individualised assessment and multidisciplinary care planning; secondly, attempts to encourage patients/clients to participate in decisions about their care; thirdly, patterns of communication which avoid exerting power and control over patients; and fourthly, attempts to modify the environment to promote autonomy and independence and minimise risk.

Pearson et al. (1993) studied the quality of care in nursing homes. In general, residents (n = 1374) were satisfied with their care. Most liked the food (77 %) although 27 % agreed that the meals are boring. They have enough say in what they do with their time (84 %) and their family and friends are welcome (96 %). However, almost one-third thought that they cannot vary their daily routine (27 %) or that it is boring to be there (30 %).

Different personnel groups may have different attitudes to patient autonomy. Mattiasson & Andersson (1995a) found that although there was in general strong support for authentic autonomy of elderly people by staff, nurses, assistant nurses and auxiliary staff showed stronger support for the expressed will of the patient comparing to nurse aides. Nurses and nurses aides expressed stronger support for decisional autonomy than assistant nurses and auxiliary staff.

Donnelly & Anderson (1990) found that nurses were most supportive in maintaining a high degree of autonomy for patients, while the physicians were least supportive. Their study indicated that physicians, nurses and dieticians with a special interest in diabetes are supportive of their own roles, but physicians tend to see themselves being in charge of diabetes care while nurses and dieticians value patient autonomy more.

Physicians attitudes have been investigated in connection with euthanasia. For example, Howard et al. (1997) assessed how frequently physicians (n = 355) could perceive a desire for euthanasia and whether they would be willing to provide patients the same interventions. They found that most physicians would make decisions for patients that correlate with decisions they would make for themselves. In addition, many physicians make decisions for patients that reflect patient autonomy, even when the physician cannot perceive the desire or need themselves.

Ende et al. (1990) assessed physicians' preferences for patient autonomy when they are patients themselves and compared this with similar data previously obtained from a patient population. They found that the physician-patients expressed significantly stronger preferences for decision-making in general, while they showed significantly less desire for information than regular patients. However, they found that physicians, as patients, preferred that their provider take the principal role as decision-maker. For both groups, decision-making preferences declined as they faced illness of increasing severity. The researchers conclude that patients, when ill, value the care and support of a provider who is willing to assume decision-making responsibility. This attitude appears to be the norm even when patient and provider are as comparable in terms of socio-economic status and medical knowledge as are pairs of physicians. Their results suggested that patients' preferences to be relieved of major decision-making responsibility are part of the phenomenology of illness and occur even when differences between patients and providers are minimised.

*Patients' wishes and needs*

Nurses generally see themselves as respecting patients' wishes. Richter et al. (1998) studied the decisions and attitudes of nurses (n = 182) in the treatment of chronically ill and old people. Out of the respondents 80 % thought that patients' wishes are extremely or very important when making decisions concerning patients' treatment. About two-thirds (68 %) would be prepared to meet the wishes of the patients. The more important patients' wishes were judged by nurses in general, the more frequently nurses chose less aggressive forms of treatment for patients.

Farrell (1991) studied how far nurses' perceptions of patients' needs correspond to patients' views of their own needs. The questionnaire study involved 30 psychiatric and 30 general patients together with their nurses. According to the results there is little evidence that individual nurses and their patients, whether psychiatric or general, agree. The author concluded that the nurses' ability to perceive patients' needs on an individual basis is consistent with other studies which suggest that nurses use stereotypes when perceiving patients' needs (e.g. Davies & Peters 1983, Drew et al. 1989, Eddington et al. 1990).

The failure to take into account patients' wishes may be due to the difficulties experienced by patients in expressing their wishes because of incapacity. However, according to Elander et al. (1993), if patients have limited capacities to be autonomous, this does not need to mean that decisions concerning all the patient's activities of daily living have to be made by caregivers. However, the fact is that taking care of hospitalised patients in long-term care involves ethical problems in different areas (e.g. Elander & Hermerén 1989).

The effects of giving patients choice and independence are highlighted in an article by Owen (1995). This article discusses new practices in nursing, which involve giving choices to elderly patients with dementia. In giving them choices (such as what foods to eat) and in giving them opportunities to socialise, some nurses have found that some of their patients have actually improved. They believe that it is possible to slow down patients' loss of ability if they are allowed choices and given independence. This demonstrates the positive effects that supporting elderly patients autonomy can have on them.

*Nursing activities*

There are certain nursing activities which are particularly common in the care of elderly patients. The WHO (1987) has published a European study of nursing care and of the planning, implementation and evaluation of care provided by nurses in 11 countries in the European region. The data were collected from 707 elderly persons aged 65 years and over. It was found that out of 24 categories of needs, skin care, hygiene and body movement were ranked above other needs related to the patients' diagnosis. In general, nursing care objectives were physical/physiological in nature. On average there were 2.2 planned interventions to every objective and 2.8 planned interventions to each need in elderly patients.

Activities in geriatric nursing care vary from one professional group to the next; this was ascertained in the study by Isola and Laitinen (1995). They examined data collected with a follow-up questionnaire among 197 nursing staff on two geriatric wards. The personnel spent most of their working hours delivering food to patients. Specialized nurses spent most of their time washing patients and in skin care, registered nurses spent most of their time reporting and trained nurses observing patients' condition. In all professional groups delivering food and helping patients to the toilet were the primary nursing functions.

Other studies have also concluded that the accent in geriatric nursing is on physical care. Salmon (1993) observed the interactions of 27 nurses on two psychogeriatric wards. Interactions with patients were observed in 36 % of the observations. Of these interactions, 80 % were concerned with physical care such as meals, medication and dressing. Overall, 33 % of the interactions were positive, i.e. informing, questioning and general conversation.

Higgs et al. (1992) interviewed elderly patients (n = 291) on long-term wards, focusing on the degree of choice which patients felt they had in relation to daily activities. Eighty per cent of the elderly patients interviewed expressed satisfaction with their own level of personal autonomy. However, 46 % experienced loss of independence, which was the worst thing about being admitted to a long-term care facility.

Patients' and nurses' perceptions of daily activities may differ. Jang (1992) studied both patient and staff perceptions of the autonomy of institutionalised elderly patients, particularly in relation to their daily activities. The findings indicated that residents' choices over daily activities of importance to them might not have matched those of staff.

*Patients' nutrition and feeding*

Everyday nursing practice involves a wide range of ethical conflicts that have to do with autonomy. Problems in the health care environment with old age increase the likelihood of participation in ethical problem-solving; these include treatment choices, advance directives, living wills, termination of treatment, and decisions associated with nutrition and hydration (Pinch & Parsons 1997). Mattiasson and Andersson (1995b) also give examples of conflicts emerging in everyday practice: freedom of movement, choice of food, what to wear and so on. For the nursing home patient with diminished autonomy, solutions to these problems are crucial because of their impact on the quality of the patient's daily life. As Tschudin (1986) believes, many of our day-to-day choices and decisions in nursing practice are ethical in nature.

Sidenvall et al. (1994) studied patients' meals in geriatric care with respect to both the intentions of nursing staff and patients' assessments, and with respect to patients' experiences and the extent to which they expected to be able to influence the meal situation as regards behaviour and table manners, eating competence and diet. Mentally oriented patients (n = 18) and their primary enrolled nurses (n = 21) took part in this study. On the basis of the results, both patients and nursing staff aimed to create as natural and independent a meal situation as possible. Lack of communication was reported as a problem by nursing staff, and they had to ask patients' opinion all the time.

In addition, the choice of diet was found problematic in some cases. The patients felt they were unable to reach their own standards of behaviour at the table and found it difficult to eat in the dining room at the beginning of their hospital stay. In addition, the elderly patients did not expect to be able to influence the menus on the ward. Out of 21 patients, 16 did not participate in deciding on their own menu, and two said they made choices regarding breakfast. Differences were also observed between the perceptions of patients and nurses with regard to the elderly patients' eating competence and collective eating.

When aged patients enter the terminal phase, spoon-feeding becomes difficult. When patients with incurable dementia diseases no longer take food or fluid voluntarily, nurses have to make the decision on whether or not to force feed patients (e.g. Bexell et al. 1985.) Patients who refuse or lose all interest in food and drink may cause difficult ethical problems (Watson 1993), particularly so in the case of terminally demented elderly (Nordberg & Athlin 1989). Åkerlund and Nordberg (1985) interviewed nurses (n = 40) about their experiences of feeding severely demented patients. They found that nurses felt a demand to keep patients alive, while they stressed the patients' right to act autonomously. These nurses felt anxious and they were unsure how to make the correct judgement with regard to feeding demented patients (also Norberg et al. 1980a,b.) On the other hand, Norberg et al. (1988) found in their study in 23 nursing homes in Sweden that nursing personnel were not able to differentiate between a patient's loss of will to eat and a patient's inability to eat. Watson (1994) has also stated that decisions about whether or not to continue with feeding in the terminal stages should not be left solely to nursing staff.

Nursing staff have different views on patients' autonomy with regard to feeding. Mattiasson & Andersson (1994) investigated the personal attitudes of nursing home staff and their experience of coping with rational nursing home patients who refused to eat and drink (n = 189). Professional caregivers in 13 nursing homes and nursing home units in Sweden were asked to judge an ethical conflict involving a situation. Approximately 50 % believed that the patient's wishes regarding food refusal must be respected. Nursing aides were over represented among those not supporting the patients' wishes, i.e. they tended to support patients' autonomy less than the other professionals.

Nurses working in different areas have different perceptions of eating problems. This was found in the study by Kuuppelomäki and Lauri (1989) on nurses' (n = 40) decision-making and their perceptions of eating problems with the elderly, seriously demented patients and with old cancer patients in terminal care. Nurses were interviewed after they had read a vignette describing a situation where an old patient refused to eat. Most nurses in cancer care did not want to feed patients against their will, while in dementia care, most nurses were prepared to do so.

Different professional groups may have different attitudes and role perceptions as to patients' feeding problems. Watts et al. (1986) found that nurses in the United States preferred the tube feeding option compared with physicians. Wilson (1992) found that the patient's physician was the major agent initiating decisions to tube feed. The physicians' dominant role was largely a consequence of their power to initiate tube feeding. The patients' charts reflected limited interaction between the physician and other involved persons, including family members and other health care professionals. Documentation (n = 10) indicated that a nurse was involved in the decision to initiate tube feeding in one instance only. Eight of the ten tube fed patients were unable to provide their written or expressed consent, as they had been deemed incompetent at the time tube feeding was initiated. Documented decisions made by physicians and family members do not reflect whether or not they were carrying out patients' wishes (Wilson 1992).

Day et al. (1995) studied nurses' (40 cancer nurses and 40 dementia nurses) attitudes to patients' artificial feeding using vignettes followed by semi-structured interviews. They found that 42 nurses would not feed the competent terminal cancer patient, and most based their decisions on the patient's right to refuse treatment, a concept inherent in autonomy. Of the 40 dementia nurses, 73 % would attempt feeding while 27 % would not. Those who would not feed most often indicated autonomy and quality of life as principles underlying their decisions.

## Dressing

Clothes play an important role in preserving identity and asserting an individual's uniqueness. It has been suggested that the provision of individual clothing is an important contribution, not only to the older person's self-respect and dignity but also to the attitudes of those providing care, by encouraging them to view the person as an individual (Meredith 1987, Burgess et al. 1988). Elander & Hermerén (1989) found that paternalistic behaviour by personnel included actions to the effect that the patients must not participate in decisions concerning how they are dressed.

In Mattiasson & Andersson's (1995a) case study, the patient's wish to dress herself did not seem unreasonable to the staff. Nursing home staff showed a positive attitude to helping the patient execute her autonomous decision (i.e. support decisional autonomy). However, lack of staff may prevent caregivers from spending as much time as necessary enquiring into the patient's preferences. Time most often sets the limit for letting the patient exercise even decisional (i.e. partial) autonomy.

## Cultural issues

In a study of the attitudes of elderly subjects from different ethnic groups towards patient autonomy in medical decision-making, Blackhall et al. (1995) surveyed 800 Korean-American, Mexican-American, African-American and white European-American patients. They found that ethnicity was the primary factor related to attitude towards truth-telling and patient decision-making. Korean Americans and Mexican Americans were significantly less likely than European Americans and African Americans to believe that a patient should be told the diagnosis of metastatic cancer. Korean and Mexican Americans were less likely than African and European Americans to believe that a patient should be told of a terminal prognosis and less likely to believe that the patient should make decisions about the use of life-supporting technology. Instead, Korean and Mexican Americans tended to believe that the family should make decisions about the use of life support. Further, Mexican Americans with more years of education were more likely to believe that the patient should be told the diagnosis. In the European American group, Protestants were more likely than non-Protestants to believe that the patient should be told about a terminal prognosis and were more likely to believe that the patient should be the primary decision-maker. However, socioeconomic status did not predict attitudes in the European and African American patients.

The meaning of the concept of autonomy also varies across cultures. Katzko et al. (1998) examined the self-concept of the elderly in a cross-cultural perspective using an open-ended sentence completion methodology. The results revealed, firstly, differences which reflected an individualistic (Dutch) vs. collectivistic (Spanish) distinction between the two cultures. Secondly, the notion of meaningful ageing was interpreted differently.

Ethical problems are often of a similar nature in different countries. This was found in an interview study with nurses in Sweden and England (Elander et al. 1993). However, ethical reasoning may also vary among nurses in different counties. Nordberg et al. (1994) interviewed 149 registered nurses in seven countries concerning their reasoning on whether or not to feed severely demented patients. They found that nurses in Australia, Canada and Sweden most often chose not to feed demented patients, while nurses in Arizona, California, Finland and Israel often selected to feed the patient as their first choice. Although the justifications varied, the reasons to feed patients were related to the ethical principle of sanctity of life, beneficence (or love and loyalty in China). Those whose first choice was to withdraw feeding gave a high rank to the ethical principle of autonomy.

There are cultural differences in feeding terminal patients (see Watson 1994). Nordberg and Hirschfeld (1987) found that Scandinavian caregivers felt that the prolongation of unnecessary suffering was to be avoided, while nurses in Israel felt that the prolongation of life was an obligation. In an exploratory, open-ended, and non-random study, 60 health care workers in nine long-term care institutions in Israel were questioned regarding their experiences, thoughts and feelings related to force feeding senile demented patients. Israeli care workers' actions as well as their emotional reactions seemed the logical outcome of Jewish sanctity of life ethics: patients were force fed and caregivers did not feel guilty for using force or accepting suffering, since they felt obliged to preserve life and thus their actions were right (Norberg & Hirshfeld 1987).

### 5.3 Autonomy and acute care

As well as discussing aspects of patient autonomy in acute care, the text below also reviews studies on nursing activities in surgical care, issues relating to patients, DNR orders and traumatology.

In a WHO study (1987) on nursing activities in surgical care, the data were collected from 4477 surgical patients between ages 15 and 65. It was found that the day before operation, emotion/feeling needs were reported most frequently as needs of nursing care among surgical patients. Need for adaptation, hygiene and sleep/rest were also frequently recorded. For days 2 and 3, hygiene, ingestion/digestion and circulation came out at the top of the list. There were almost 20 nursing care objectives per patient, six out of ten were related to physical/physiological objectives. Nurses intervened for the patient most often, and carried out educational/information-giving interventions second.

*Do-not-resuscitate decisions*

Nurses working in different environments may have different views on who would be best able to support the patients' autonomy in Do-Not-Resuscitate (DNR) decisions. In a study by Marchette et al. (1993) it was found that compared to nurses working in a private non-profit hospital, nurses working in the Veterans Administration Medical Center felt more often that family members would be best placed to support the patient's autonomy in DNR decisions. This may be due to the fact that long-term care stresses decisions made by the patient and family members, while fewer critical care patients than long-term care patients are able to speak and make their DNR wishes known.

Health care personnel may have different views on what is important and how they actually behave in care. Ott (1986) studied the support given by nurses for patient autonomy in DNR decisions by asking 251 critical care nurses to read four descriptions of hypothetical patients with a terminal and irreversible health condition. They were asked to choose the agent who could best support patient autonomy in each situation. After reading four descriptions, the nurse selected the person who could best support patient autonomy. However, when asked to select the person whose opinion would be regarded as most appropriate should the situation occur, many selected the physician. According to this study there is a discrepancy between who nurses think should and who actually does make the DNR decision.

Mello & Jenkinson (1998) compared decision-making practices concerning DNR orders in British and American hospitals. A total of 34 physicians and nurses in one American and one British hospital were interviewed about their decision-making practices. Qualitative methods of data analysis were employed. The study revealed that while the American and British hospitals had adopted similar formal protocols for DNR decision-making, in practice the British physicians often made DNR decisions unilaterally, whereas the American physicians sought the patient's or surrogate's consent in every instance, even where it was not legally required. The British decision-making model enables physicians to reduce the inappropriate use of resuscitation, but at the expense of patient autonomy. In contrast, the American approach fully respects patient autonomy, but except in cases of medical futility grants physicians no authority to refuse to render treatments that are in their judgment contraindicated.

The attitudes of Swedish cardiologists and nurses regarding information given to patients and relatives concerning DNR status were surveyed by Lofmark & Nilstun (1998). Data were collected using questionnaires in nationwide settings. A 10 % random sample of members of the Swedish Cardiac Society, 104 physicians and 196 nurses participated in the study. According to most Swedish cardiologists and cardiac nurses, patients and relatives should be honestly informed about a patient's DNR status if they ask for information. Almost all (97 %) answered that the relatives of a non-competent patient should be informed when they ask and two-thirds (67 %) believe that the relatives should be informed even if they do not ask. Most of the respondents (61 %) said that the patient, if mentally competent, should be informed about the DNR status first and decide if the information should be passed on to relatives. Only 12 % of the respondents were of the opinion that if the relatives asked for this information to be withheld from the patient, this should be respected even if the patient asked for information, and 45 % believed it should be respected if the patient did not ask. With reference to the latter, many (31 %) were uncertain. The cardiologists and cardiac nurses expressed almost identical opinions in the matter of informing patients and relatives about DNR status. More training in informing patients and relatives about delicate matters is probably required, together with more knowledge about the wishes of very ill patients.

*Experiences of autonomy*

Mazaux et al. (1997) assessed which social activities were still impaired five years after a traumatic brain injury (TBI) in adults at hospital or at their homes, and which neuropsychological impairments were associated with this loss of social autonomy. This was a cross-sectional study of 79 patients selected by convenience sampling from the follow-up cohort of an epidemiological survey of 2,116 TBI patients. Up to 16 patients suffered disability for at least one social skill because of cognitive/behavioural reasons. Seven needed full-time supervision. Performing administrative tasks and financial management, writing letters and calculating, driving, planning the week, and using public transport were the most impaired social abilities. Loss of social autonomy was mainly observed in severely injured patients. Univariate analysis showed that mental fatigability, motor slowing, memory difficulties, and disorders of executive function were associated with low scores on the GOS, unemployment, and difficulties in shopping, using public transport, and performing financial management and administrative tasks.

There are different personality types which may influence how a person experiences his or her autonomy. McWilliam et al. (1994) found that patients (n = 21) with a positive mindset felt their autonomy was not threatened even when cared for in a paternalistic manner. This suggests the need to make an assessment of an individual's personality type in considering how best to promote his or her autonomy and independence.

Williams et al. (1998) applied self-determination theory to explore the motivational basis of adherence to long-term medication prescriptions. Adult outpatients with various diagnoses who had been on medication for at least one month and who expected to continue (a) completed questionnaires that assessed their autonomous regulation, other motivation variables, and perceptions of their physicians' support of their autonomy by hearing their concerns and offering choice; (b) provided subjective ratings of their adherence and a two-day retrospective pill count during an interview with a clinical psychologist; and (c) provided a 14-day prospective pill count during a subsequent, brief telephone survey. LISREL analyses supported the self-determination model for adherence by confirming that patients' autonomous motivation for adherence did mediate the relationship between patients' perceptions of their physicians' autonomy support and their own medication adherence.

The purpose of Niedz's (1998) study was to examine hospital patients' perceptions of service quality in relation to four independent variables: (a) nurses' perceptions of human resource practices, (b) nurses' perceptions of autonomy in practice, (c) patient satisfaction with nursing care, and (d) patients' perceptions of organisational climate for service. The sample consisted of 102 nurse-patient dyads in an acute care hospital. Patients responded to the Modified Health Care Service Performance

Instrument, the revised LaMonica-Oberst Patient Satisfaction Scale, and the Organizational Climate for Service Semantic Differential. Nurses responded to the Employee Turnover Diagnostic and the Dempster Practice Behaviors Scale. Patient satisfaction with nursing care and patients' perceptions of organisational climate for service were both positively related to patients' perceptions of service quality.

*5.4 Autonomy in gynaecological and maternity care*

Ethical issues related to gynaecological and maternity care are quite extensively discussed in the literature. Specifically, studies have dealt with genetic counselling (Headings 1997, White 1998), moral issues regarding mothers who use drugs (DeVille & Kopelman 1998), and mothers' illness, pregnancy and decisions concerning the health of the foetus (e.g. Iseminger & Lewis 1998). Ethics in obstetrics and gynaecology (Chervenak & McCullogh 1997) and the practice of obstetric ultrasound have received special attention (Chervenak & McCullough 1993a). Another concern has been with how beneficence and respect for autonomy could interact in obstetrics and gynaecology practices (Chervenak & McCullough 1998a,b), how to identify and manage ethical conflicts in the gynaecologist-patient relationship (Chervenak & McCullough 1993b) and how to improve patients' decision-making in the case of hysterectomy (Gambone & Reiter 1997). It has been recognised that a humane childbirth is an issue of respect for women's autonomy and the degree of decision-making allowed to her by the system in which she gives birth (Crafter & Rowan 1998, Mander 1998). However, studies concerning the autonomy of mothers or gynaecological patients are rare.

Wertz and Fletcher (1998) studied geneticists' attitudes to prenatal sex selection. They have conducted an extensive survey of geneticists in 37 nations to measure their attitudes to prenatal sex selection (2903 geneticists and genetic counsellors). The study showed that 29 % would perform prenatal diagnosis for a couple with four girls who wanted a boy and would abort a female fetus. In all, 47 % had requests for sex selection.

Kim et al. (1998) studied the desire of patients to know whether trainees would be taking part in their care. Questionnaires were sent out to women (n = 111) who had undergone elective hysterectomies at two teaching hospitals. The specific concern was with women's awareness of and attitudes towards the participation of residents and medical students in their care and with how they thought physicians should communicate information regarding residents to patients. Thirty-seven (63 %, n = 59) of the patients knew that a resident had been involved in their care. Eighty percent of the respondents felt it important to know how residents were supervised and what they would do during the operation. Nearly half did not know whether a medical student had been involved in their care. Over 90 % agreed that the attending gynaecologist should tell patients that a resident would participate in the operation and what the resident would do. Most believed that residents are adequately supervised and that medical students have time to provide more attention to patients. They concluded that open discussions can promote patient autonomy, maintain public confidence in academic health institutions, and benefit future patients.

Data on patients' experiences at a gynaecology outpatient department were collected between 1988 and 1992 by 252 spontaneous letters (Lang & Nikkonen 1994).

According to the results, 68 % of women's statements concerned the personnel's activities. The subjects of the perceptions were divided into three categories: patient-personnel relationship (40 %), waiting time (39 %) and information (21 %). The following aspects of care were valued by the patients: individuality, privacy, self-determination, kindness, safety, objectivity, and efficiency.

There have also been studies to compare childbirth experiences in different cultures: Finnish Lutherans (n = 32), Canadian Orthodox Jews (n = 30) and American Mormons (n = 60). All the mothers considered it useful that they are taught how to look after themselves during pregnancy. Women in Finland have faith in the maternity hospital, but do not expect to receive much medical assistance in labour. Finnish and American mothers are reluctant simply to follow the advice of experts, but they feel they have relevant knowledge themselves on how to act. Finnish women (82.5 %) decide independently whether or not to follow the instructions given, 60 % say they take the initiative in their own care. The vast majority (95 %) were of the opinion that maternity care should be based on a joint agreement between the mothers, midwife and doctors. Almost all attached much importance to having the opportunity actively to participate and to choose between different treatments. Almost all also wanted to know the details relating to childbirth and three-quarters (75 %) wanted to intervene in procedures taken during delivery. The mothers were also reluctant to submit to standard hospital routines. Women in Finland and the US took a more active role in childbirth than Canadian Orthodox Jews (Vehviläinen-Julkunen et al. 1994).

The connections between self-determination, nursing practice and the nursing environment were evaluated by 476 mothers in two Finnish hospitals. It was found that mothers have wishes which they wanted to be realised during labour. Before delivery, 80 % believed they would be able to decide independently on matters relating to their delivery. Similarly, 80 % were willing to get pain relief during labour. However, almost one-fifth (19 %) said they had not received the pain relief they would have wanted to. Sixteen per cent were of the opinion that they had decided on their treatment during delivery; 34 % thought that the decisions had been made by the midwife; and 2 % that they were made by the medical doctor. Almost one-third or 30 % would be willing to take a more active part in decision-making in future deliveries. On the other hand, 79 % said they had been supported in decision-making at the first stage and 69 % at the second stage. In the delivery room 49 % were allowed to decide on the administration of an enema, 74 % on pain management and 55 % on treatment during the first stage. Almost half or 46 % of the mothers had been allowed to decide on their position in the second stage; at reception they had also been asked whether they would be having a support person in the delivery room (Carey & Helander 1993).

# Patient's privacy in the literature

### 1. General

A database search was carried out on Medline express using the keywords "privacy" and "patient privacy". Between 1966 and 1998, a total of 1254 abstracts have been published on related subjects. The keyword "patient privacy" produced no more than 48 hits. Manual analysis of the abstracts and publications revealed a greater number of empirical studies in this field; these are listed under the references.

The concept of privacy pertains to all areas of human activity in society. It appears in the literature of several different disciplines, including psychology, sociology, anthropology, political science, law, architecture, and the design professions. According to Rawnsley (1980), privacy may be described as a psychosocial reality that exists within a matrix of political, technological, psychological and evolutionary phenomena.

Westin (1970), by contrast, says that the origin of man's need for privacy probably lies in his animal origins, and that men and animals share several basic mechanisms for claiming privacy among their own fellows. Virtually all animals seek periods of individual seclusion or small-group intimacy. This is usually described as the tendency towards territoriality, in which an organism lays private claim to an area of land, water, or air and defends it against intrusion by members of its own species. Westin also describes the concept of privacy in primitive societies and in political systems. He seems to concentrate on the disclosure of data, (1970, 7) calling privacy "the claim of individuals, groups, or institutions to determine for themselves when, how, and to what extent information is communicated to others".

Privacy is also recognised as one of the important concepts in nursing (e.g. Yura & Walsh 1988). There are several vulnerable and intimate situations in which the nurse may invade the patient's privacy (e.g. Bäck & Wikblad 1998). Rawnsley (1980) refers to a relevant responsibility for nursing, because of nurses care for their clients during many intimate and vulnerable moments.

There exists no single, universal definition for the concept of privacy. In 1970, Westin observed that there were few values so fundamental to society as privacy that have been left so undefined in social theory or that have been the subject of such vague and confused writing. Other researchers have also pointed at the difficulties of defining the concept of privacy (Younger 1972, MacCormick 1974, Schuster 1976a, Velecky 1978, Young 1978a,b, Burgoon 1982, Gifford 1987, Bauer 1994).

There has not been very much empirical research into privacy, particularly in the fields of health care and nursing. Some work was done in the field of environment psychology during the 1960s and 1970s, when according to Schuster (1976a) the literature dealing with privacy increased sixfold; a similar trend can be identified later as well (Burgoon 1982). More recently, privacy has mainly been discussed in connection with information technology (e.g. Eliasson & Poropatich 1998, Moehr 1998), genetics (e.g. Hendricks 1997, Weaver 1997, Deftos 1998), research ethics (e.g. Horner 1998) and the care of AIDS/HIV patients (e.g. Etzioni 1998).

In the 1970s, Ingham (1978) listed some reasons for the scarcity of research evidence; almost two decades later, Bauer (1994) shares the same thoughts: There is a logical problem in investigating a personal area that by its nature is closed to scrutiny. As Gifford (1987, 201) observes, "in order to study privacy behaviour by field observation, the investigator is almost forced to violate the subject's privacy". Data collection relies upon honesty. The researcher has to be sure that social desirability response bias does not threaten the results. Ethical issues are another reason for either not conducting the research at all or for not using confidential results.

Burden (1998, 16) is sharply critical of the research that has been done in privacy issues in nursing and midwifery: "Throughout the authors fail to define privacy nor do they identify the parameters of the problem". Psychology and sociology, she says, have contributed much more to the understanding of the concept of privacy, especially through research into related concepts of personal space and crowding.

## 2. The concept of privacy

The term "privacy" derives from the Latin words "Privatus" (Curtin 1981) and "privo", meaning "to deprive" (Rawnsley 1980). Its original usage, according to Rawnsley (1980, see also Funk 1950) was the military term private, which literally meant "to be deprived of status or rank". The stem of privacy is priv, the same as in the word privilege, which means a "favouring opportunity". In 1702, Kersey (according   to Rawnsley 1980) defined private as "particular" or "secrete", privilege as "a private or particular law".

In English-language dictionaries, privacy is defined as "withdrawal from public view or company" and "one's private life" (Webster's New World Dictionary 1986). Some researchers (e.g. Hallborg 1986) stress the aspect of freedom from the observation of other persons. One of the earliest legal analyses of the concept of privacy was presented by Warren and Brandeis (1890). Their focus was on the question of whether the existing law affords a principle which can properly be invoked to protect the privacy of the individual; and if it does, what the nature and extent of such protection is. They say that common law secures to each individual the right of determining, ordinarily, to what extent his thoughts, sentiments, and emotions shall be communicated to others.

Privacy emphasises the individuality of human beings. Historically (see e.g. Markova 1995), particularly Kantian ethics, the idea of human dignity was a culmination of the perspective of individualism that had been nurtured in European culture for two or three centuries. Two main sources of the individualistic perspective have been identified in scholarly analyses of individualism. The first of these emphasises the role of factors in the socio-economic-cultural sphere of ordinary life. The second source of individualism was to be found in the Renaissance philosophy, science and art, contained in the idea that the individual is a free agent responsible for his or her own fate. In individualism, there are also negative sides, which are realised in the total withdrawal of human beings from social life (Doyal 1997).

## 2.1 Perspectives in concept descriptions

Several authors have proposed their definitions for the concept of privacy. In a review on privacy and communication, Burgoon (1982) has made a distinction between six analytic perspectives in the literature. These perspectives provide the structure for the present chapter.

Analytic perspectives to the concept of privacy are as follows (based on Burgoon 1982):

- Units experiencing privacy: single persons — group
- Desired — achieved
- Prerequisites — actual experience
- Reactive — proactive
- Human responsibility — legal basis: privacy as a right
- Typologies with different foundations: degrees, states, level of publicity, territorial enroachment, needs

Definitions of the concept of privacy differ according to the unit experiencing the privacy: the unit can be either an individual or a group, or both. Altman (1975), for example, defines the units of privacy as person-to-person, person-to-group, group-to-person and group-to-group. Westin (1970, also Altman 1976, empirically tested by Marshall 1974) speaks about the desires of single persons.

Definitions of privacy can be described (see Altman 1975) either as ideal, desired state or actual end state realised. Desired privacy is a subjective statement of an ideal level of interaction with others, of how much or how little contact is desired at any given moment. Achieved privacy is the actual degree of contact that results from interaction with others. If the desired privacy is equal to the achieved privacy, then there exists an optimum state of privacy.

Prerequisites and the actual experience of privacy constitute another relevant perspective. The reactive-proactive perspective can be identified, for instance, in distinctions between the emphasis on seclusion or withdrawal from interaction, and the notions of control and freedom of choice (Altman 1975, 1976). Privacy is an interpersonal boundary-control process, which paces and regulates interaction with others. It also is a dialectic process, which involves both a restriction and seeking of interaction (see Simmel 1950, Westin 1970, Altman 1975). It can be described as an input and output process: people and groups attempt to regulate contacts coming from others and outputs they make to others (Altman 1975), or it can be seen as an optimising process: there is an optimal degree of desired access of the self to others at any moment in time (see also Westin 1970, Altman 1975).

Many studies (e.g. Wolfe 1978, Colette 1984, Kerr 1985, Magaziner 1988) have employed Altman's (1975) concept of privacy, emphasising the aspect of control. This is a rather comprehensive definition in which the accent is on the subject's decision to deny as well as to grant access: privacy "is a selective control of access to the self or to one's group" (Altman 1975, 18, see also Bauer 1994). There may be two aspects of control (Wolfe 1978): first, there is the control of communication with other people, the second is controlling information/knowledge about oneself. In other words, this is a question of selective control of access to self (Altman 1975). Control of knowledge is an important part of privacy and the decision as to what information is given and what is not, or what personal information is shared with others (also Velecky 1978). This perspective can also be identified in the definition put forward by the British Medical Association (1995), according to which privacy is a fundamental right which allows individuals to decide on the manner and extent to which information about themselves is shared with others. Such personal control lies at the very core of legislation, enabling patient access to health records and reports. Regulation of personal information is also central to the definition of privacy proposed by Ziporyn (1984) and Muyskens (1982). Beardsley (1971) speaks about selective disclosure.

Privacy can also be seen as a human responsibility. This aspect is highlighted in discussions of privacy as a right of human beings (e.g. Westin 1970, Benn 1971, van den Haag 1971, Velecky 1978, Muyskens 1982, Ziporyn 1984, Barron 1990, Aiken & Catalano 1994, Bandman & Bandman 1995, British Medical Association 1995, Szekely et al. 1996, Doyal 1997). Hallborg (1986), for instance, says that the right to privacy can be inferred from the human right to freedom, making a distinction between legal right and moral right (see also e.g. Rawnsley 1980). In line with most nursing researchers, Velecky (1978) makes a strong case for moral privacy. On occasions, however, public interest may override the privacy of the individual, but in such instances the facts must be subject to close scrutiny as to whether there is a genuine necessity for disclosure (British Medical Association 1995). In the nursing context the right to freedom from interference by others involves the right to freedom from medical intervention when patients have declined treatment; of course patients also have the right to be heard and to have their beliefs respected. The right to privacy is also set out in the Patients Bill of Rights (1973, 5th item): "The patient has a right to every consideration of his privacy concerning his own medical care program."

The right to privacy places the power of disclosure in the hands of the individual. If the individual wishes to disclose any information concerning his or her health or attitudes or actions, this is his or her prerogative. If he or she authorises disclosure of information, then doing so is not a breach of confidence. But disclosure without such authorisation is prima facie wrong (Muyskens 1982.) The right to privacy has also been described as a personal right: it applies to the individual and does not extend to family members or businesses (Aiken & Catalano 1994).

The right to privacy is a crucial autonomy right. However, it is not an absolute right, and it may be overridden. This does not mean that due regard is not given to these important autonomy rights (Bandman & Bandman 1995).

Different typologies have been applied in the description of privacy. Westin (1967), for example, speaks about degrees of privacy (see also van den Haag 1971). The degrees of privacy are closely connected with the social nature of the concept (see Ingham 1978, Rawnsley 1980). The first state is called solitude and represents the popular notion of privacy. It describes the individual's separation from the group and his freedom from observation. Solitude is the most complete state of privacy an individual can achieve. The second state, intimacy, refers to the seclusion of pairs or small groups to achieve either maximally personal relationships or maximally efficient working conditions. Intimacy can result in relaxed relations or tiring hostilities. Anonymity is the state where the individual is in a public place and free from personal identification. The fourth state is the creation of psychological barriers and is called reserve. It involves limitation of communication, but it is not an isolated (Simmel 1971) or negative freedom (McCloskey 1971).

Drawing on a phenomenological study with 21 recently-hospitalised adults in the United States, Schuster (1976a) identified the following aspects of privacy: 1) privacy of life style, 2) privacy of event and 3) privacy of personality. Privacy of life style refers to the individual's preference in day-to-day living; it is quite consistent and unaltered by passage of time. Privacy of event means that for a specific activity privacy is necessary (e.g. have the door closed during showering). Privacy of personality is not transient in duration, and entails what is the innermost part of self and the domain of autonomous activity.

Privacy is a situational concept which varies across cultures. Laufer & Wolfe (1977) describe the structural aspect of the theory as situational perspective. They describe the elements of situations that must be taken into account in order to understand the individual's perception and experience of privacy and invasions of privacy. These elements are combined into three dimensions; environmental, interpersonal and self-ego dimensions. The environmental dimension includes cultural, socio-physical and life cycle elements. The interpersonal dimension includes interaction management and information management.

Gafo (1994) says that in traditional cultures, information was regulated by customs rather than formal rules, and more delicate information was transmitted by word of mouth to relatives and friends. Nowadays, however, medical reports are stored in computers, which increases the risk of access and diffusion among authorised persons. Societies in which the accent is placed on privacy, also attach much importance to autonomy, for two main reasons: first, because they feel it is the individuals who must shape their lives, on the condition that they cause no pain to others; and second, because they feel that general well-being is encouraged if the individual can have his or her own options and private matters.

## 2.2 Dimensions of the concept of privacy

The different dimensions of the concept of privacy have also been defined in different ways (e.g. Burgoon 1982, Parrott et al. 1989). A useful classification for the purposes of nursing is summarised in Figure 5.

### Physical privacy

Physical privacy is the degree to which one is physically accessible to others. That assessment is fundamentally based on subjective views. It may also be a situational assessment and liable to change in different physical environments. Physical privacy has to do with concepts of personal space and especially with the concept of territoriality. In many studies privacy is either closely related to these concepts, or personal space is described as a precondition for privacy. Lane (1990) concludes that although studies have dealt with personal space and territoriality, only a limited number address these concepts in the context of health care. There has been only very limited research into patients' experiences in response to nurses being in their proximity (Kerr 1982, Lane 1990). Gafo (1994) describes the concept of privacy as a highly complex one, physical isolation being part of it.

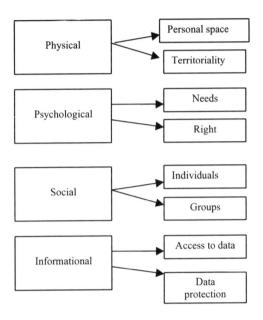

**Figure 5.** Dimensions of the concept of privacy

The concept of personal space has its roots in etiological research to study the natural life and habits of animals. A number of articles and books were published on the concept in the 1960s (e.g. Hall 1959, Little 1965, Sommer 1969), providing a solid foundation for later work. One of the earliest publications employing the concept of personal space is the work by Hall (1959), who defined personal space as the distance between people and people's preferences. According to Sommer (1969), personal space is an invisible place surrounding the human body, an individual area separating people from one another. It serves as a kind of protection zone. Insel (1978, also Meisenheimer 1982) describes personal space as a portable bubble which consciously surrounds the individual, providing a margin of safety and security.

Altman (1975) defines personal space as an invisible boundary surrounding the self; intrusion into this space creates tension or discomfort. He describes the properties of personal space by saying that it is "attached" to the self, that it is carried everywhere one goes, whereas the notion of territory usually implies a fixed, geographically immobile region (see also Little 1965). Personal-space regulation is a dynamic process that permits differential access to the self as situations change. When someone crosses a personal-space boundary, anxiety or stress often results, or even flight and aggression. Altman & Vinsel (1977) have analysed studies into privacy, some of which have been conducted in laboratories and some in everyday environments. According to these studies, intrusions into personal space-boundary may cause stress, unpleasant feelings, personal hurt and withdrawals.

Different factors are related to personal space. These include (Altman 1975) age and developmental processes, personal abnormality (socio-emotional disorders, such as those suffered by psychotics, neurotics, drug addicts), reactions to those with abnormalities, personality (extroverts-introverts, anxiety-level), sex (males have larger personal-space zones and people generally maintain greater distance form males than from females), cultural factors, interpersonal relations (friends, relatives) and situational determinants (only a few studies: formality or informality of settings, familiarity or strangeness of situations, and different places).

In most studies privacy has been defined as consisting primarily of territoriality. Territoriality refers to a physical place such as the home, office or a place in an official building (e.g. a hospital); sometimes it has also been used to refer to a certain knowledge area or social status (Pluckhan 1968, Proshansky et al. 1970, Altman 1975, Levy-Leboyer 1982). Furthermore, it has been used to describe states characterised by possessiveness, control, and authority over an area of physical space (Roberts 1978).

The concept of territory combines the physical place and the behaviour of human beings; territories are used in order to regulate collaboration and to maintain social order. Territory gives the person the opportunity to be alone in his or her territory (Proshansky et al. 1970, Edney 1974, Trierweiler 1978, Levy-Leboyer 1982).

Lyman and Scott (1967) make a distinction between public territories, home territories, interactional territories and body territories. Public territories are those areas where the individual has freedom of access, but not necessarily of action, by virtue of his or her claim to citizenship. Home territories are areas where the regular participants have a relative freedom of behaviour and a sense of intimacy and control over the area. Interactional territories refer to any area where a social gathering may occur, and body territories include the space encompassed by the human body and the anatomical space of the body. There are three types of territorial encroachment (Lyman & Scott 1967): violation, invasion and contamination. Violation is unwarranted use of the territory, invasion of territory occurs when those not entitled to entrance or use nevertheless cross the boundaries and interrupt or change the social meaning of the territory. Contamination of a territory, then, requires that it be rendered impure with respect to its definition and usage.

In nursing, Cooper (1984, see also Johnson 1979) has described the concepts of Lyman and Scott (1967) from the point of view of chronically institutionalised individuals. She suggests that territoriality can be measured by determining the prevalence and degree of the following behaviours: 1) attempting to consistently sit in the same area or chair, 2) arranging concrete boundaries around one's body, 3) rearranging body position to face away from others, 4) avoiding eye contact, 5) sitting side-by-side vs face-to-face, 6) increased sleeping or retreat into drugs, fantasies, etc and 7) various adornments of the body. All these are relevant for nursing.

Territoriality has also been described as a need (e.g. Oland 1978, Roberts 1978, Tate 1980, Hayter 1981). Yura and Walsh (1988, 94), for example, define territoriality as the possession of a prescribed area of space or knowledge that a person denotes as one's own, over which the person maintains control, defends if necessary, and receives acknowledgement from others of the identification of this space as owned. For the need of territoriality to be fully met, the person must be in control of some space, able to establish rules for the space and defend it against invasion or misuse by others, and his right to do those things must be acknowledged by other persons. Territoriality serves four functions by Hayter (1981): it provides security, privacy, autonomy and self-identity. One's own territory contributes to a feeling of relaxation and ease which is important for well-being; it also provides emotional release. She also describes the association with autonomy and defines autonomy as control of oneself and what happens to oneself. In one's own territory, a person may feel free to ask questions, resist a course of action suggested or hold out for what he or she wants, while the same person outside his territory may be submissive and withdrawn.

Among the various factors influencing territoriality (Hayter 1981), those that are particularly relevant to nursing are age, sex, health status and culture. Old persons have a strong need for a space of their own, while males seem to need more space than females. She also makes a suggestion for the assessment of territoriality and guidelines for meeting territoriality needs.

Territory is often marked by the person. The marking takes place, for example, by using personal things; others will usually show respect for the marked place (Pluckhan 1968, Altman 1975, Johnson 1979, Nelson & Paluck 1980, Levy-Leboyer 1982). In hospital, territory may be marked by different personal belongings (see Hovi 1990).

Territoriality has been analysed in the context of the physical environment (Williams 1988, also Reizenstein 1982), most clearly so in the nursing literature on the care of the elderly (e.g. Johnson 1979). Researchers have also developed an instrument for determining client perceptions in response to space intrusions (Lane 1990). In general, however, the physical environment of patient care has commanded only limited attention among nurse researchers (Williams 1988). The issue of privacy has been addressed primarily in surveys in which patients have been asked preferences about single, double, or multibed rooms. Thompson and Goldin (1975), for example, concluded that this issue would always remain an open question. In the study by Wood (1977, see also Campbell 1984) the purpose was to determine whether there were differences in sensory disturbances between patients randomly assigned to single and two-bed rooms. Reduced sensory stimulation and social isolation were considered probable causes for the results which revealed more disturbances among the patients in single units. Williams (1988) concludes that there is little evidence that the physical design of general medicine and surgical nursing units is the sole variable related to patients' emotional comfort or their satisfaction with nursing.

*Psychological privacy*

Psychological privacy concerns the ability of individuals to control affective and cognitive inputs and outputs, to think and form attitudes, beliefs or values, and the right to determine with whom and under what circumstances they will share thoughts and feelings or reveal intimate information (Burgoon 1982). In other words this concept is closely connected with definitions of privacy as a need or right. It is also closely connected with physical privacy: personal space and territory are also psychological concepts. Rawnsley (1980) classifies the positions of privacy as a psychological need or function into three groups: 1) those who consider privacy to be an antisocial anachronism, 2) those who think privacy is a necessary defence mechanism against pressures of society and 3) those who believe privacy to be a vital condition for personal growth.

Privacy as a need can also be psychological in nature (Sundström et al. 1982, see also Westin 1967, Ingham 1978). In Westin (1970, also Ingham 1978), we can see this in the description of the four, partly overlapping functions of privacy: 1) need for personal autonomy; we need to retain a sense of individuality, 2) it provides an opportunity for emotional release, 3) need to self-evaluation and 4) to provide or to allow limited and protected communication. Privacy needs can also be organised in a hierarchic fashion (Sundström et al. 1982). In nursing, Yura and Walsh (1988) define the need of privacy (or more exactly territoriality) as a freedom need rather than a survival and closeness need.

In her analysis of the psychological dimension of privacy and communication, Burgoon (1982) also links up the concept with the functions it performs (see also Westin 1970, Altman 1975). These have to do with the development of self-identity, self-evaluation, self-protection through control over outputs, self-protection through control over inputs, personal autonomy and personal growth. Psychological privacy can have either positive or negative meanings to all of these, developing or limiting the growth of human beings.

*Social privacy*

Social privacy includes the individual's ability and effort to control social contacts for reasons such as managing interactions or maintaining status divisions (also Westin 1970, Altman 1975, 1977). It is best understood as both an individual and a group state. For individuals, privacy seems to be necessary for individual well-being (Yura & Walsh 1988). It serves to manage social interactions and establish strategies for interacting with others (Altman 1977). Social privacy also has a strong cultural connotation (Roberts & Gregor 1971, see also Gafo 1994). Anthropologists have classified different privacy categories, and according to some studies (e.g. Hall 1959, Westin 1970, Altman 1977) culture has an impact on the concept and on the ways and means in which people try to maintain their privacy.

Among the authors who have described social privacy, Hall (1966, 1970, see also Mallon-Palmer 1980) identified four distance zones, i.e. intimate, personal, social and public. The first zone (intimate distance) covers the range of 0-18 inches. The second zone (personal distance) spans the range from 1.5 to 4 feet. This distance is the characteristic spacing people use with one another: intrusion beyond this distance is uncomfortable. The third zone (social distance-) ranges from about 4 to 12 feet and is the normal distance at which business and general social contact occur. The last zone (public distance) varies from 12 to 25 feet and is the distance at which communication cues become quite gross. There are cultural differences in these zones (Watson 1970, Altman 1975, see also Little 1965) and Leibman (1970) and Levy-Leboyer (1982), for instance, have criticized the definition of personal space based on distance zones, such as that proposed by Sommer (1969). According to them, this approach is far too mechanistic in drawing our attention to measuring distances between people. Leibman (1970), for example, emphasises that personal space is regulated by interaction and that is why it may constantly change. The need for personal space is also in constant flux: in a formal and strange environment people have a larger personal space than in a familiar, safe place.

Burgoon (1982), however, says that the four categories identified by Hall (1966, 1970) could easily be adapted to serve as categories of social privacy as well. Westin (1970) employed the categories of anonymity, reserve and intimacy, which all have to do with social privacy. Burgoon (1982, 221-222, see also Kelvin 1973) summarises the elements of social privacy as:
- control of who the participants of an interaction are
- control of the frequency of interaction
- control of the length of interaction
- control of the content of interaction.

The degree of formality in the situation also has to do with the concept of social privacy: the more formal the situation, the more reserve. Furthermore, social privacy entails being free not only from actual interaction with others, but also from any perceived pressures on one's own course of action: one has privacy to the extent that one is able to control one's own actions indirectly by controlling interactions with others (Kelvin 1973, Burgoon 1982).

*Informational privacy*

Informational privacy relates to an individual's right to determine how, when, and to what extent data about the self will be released to another person (Westin 1970) or to an organisation (such as a hospital). Although closely connected with the notion of psychological privacy, Burgoon (1982) sets it apart because informational privacy goes beyond that which is under personal control.

Informational privacy has to do with various things in society and health care. In particular, the expansion of information technology and the growing use of computers has placed growing demands on data protection  The main concern here is with the questions of who has access to the data, what its contents should include and how it should be protected.

Gafo (1994) also speaks about informational privacy. This informational dimension has to do with the non-dispersion of private information concerning persons. This is a highly controversial aspect today on account of the frequent revelations by doctors of information concerning their patients' private life against their will. Informational privacy is lost when information about a person is obtained against his or her will, be it because there is an obligation to disclose it or because it concerns an area of intimacy over which the individual wishes to retain control.

*Links with other concepts*

Privacy is most often connected with the concepts of personal space, territoriality and crowding (see the famous definition by Altman 1975, 1976). These concepts have been widely used in the later literature for describing and operationalising the concept of privacy. The concept of privacy is central, providing the glue that binds the four concepts together. Privacy is a central regulatory process by which a person (or group) makes himself more or less accessible and open to others; it is a kind of freedom to select (see also Proshansky et al. 1970, Westin 1970, Altman 1976, Schuster 1976 a,b, Hallborg 1986).

Privacy is also linked up with other concepts. Writing about the general principle of privacy, Benn (1971) suggests that it might be grounded in the more general principle of respect for persons. The second ideal to which privacy is closely connected is that of the free man in a minimally regulated society; and this conception of privacy is closely bound up with the liberal ideal. The third ideal is that of independently minded individual, whose actions are governed by his or her own principles.

In Spain, differences have been drawn between privacy and intimacy (Gafo 1994). To speak of intimacy may mean a greater affirmation of relationships among human beings; that individual fulfilment is carried out through human relationships in which privacy is converted into a means of personal dialogue. In itself privacy is a negative term: it refers to the setting up of barriers which must not be transgressed in human relationships. To speak of intimacy means to refer to the totality of contents by which the deepest nucleus of the human being is defined. Privacy can be achieved from such attitudes as indifference, even disdain towards others, while intimacy can constitute a challenge in establishing means of communication.

Increasingly the term privacy is used in connection with the concept of autonomy. Privacy has been described as an element of autonomy (Muyskens 1982), or as having close links with autonomy (Doyal 1997). As Doyal suggests, the more autonomy we exercise in our lives, the more we will benefit from privacy, and the more we benefit from privacy, the more autonomy we will possess. Privacy is not, however, synonymous with autonomy. The right to privacy is a right of limited physical and informational inaccessibility, and it can be confusing to think of this right as reducible to a right to be free to do something or a right to act autonomously. The right to privacy is a specification of and is justified by the principle of respect for autonomy, but they are not synonyms (Beauchamp & Childress 1994). The principle of confidentiality in the relationship between health professionals and clients is based on the right of privacy, which in entailed by the principle of autonomy. In her analysis of privacy and communication, Burgoon (1982) identifies the personal autonomy as one function of psychological privacy. Friedlander (1982) defines privacy as a means to achieve autonomy.

## 3. Realisation of privacy

Privacy can be realised in different forms. The discussion below describes the various factors which support and restrict the realisation of privacy. Some of these factors have already been discussed in connection with personal space and territoriality.

Expectations play an important part in the realisation of privacy. People's expectations with regard to privacy will vary according to their situation. People tend to expect the greatest degree of privacy and strictest confidentiality to be observed when they are visited in their own homes or when they see health professionals in a private consultation. In a description of privacy and human needs, Doyal (1997) makes an important point in saying that there is nothing valuable about privacy in itself unless the individuals concerned have something they want to do in private as well as the practical means to achieve it.

The realisation of privacy can be informational, psychological, social or physical in nature (see Parrott et al. 1989). Informational privacy is usually connected with the confidentiality of the personal information of clients in health care organisations (Edgar 1994, van der Leer 1994). In most countries this kind of confidentiality is protected by law and other regulations (e.g. in UK Code of Professional Conduct 1992, Data Protection Act 1998). Psychologically, the realisation of privacy is connected with the concepts of personal integrity (Edgar 1994) and dignity (Shotton & Seedhouse 1992). In social terms, the realisation of privacy is connected with relationships with other people. Physically, then, realisation is tied up with the physical environment and the opportunities to act bodily as one wants.

### 3.1 Factors supporting privacy

A distinction can be made between internal and external factors that support privacy (Figure 6).

Accounts of internal supportive factors are few and far between. However, the behavioural mechanisms of human beings have received some attention. According to Altman (1975, 1976) people attempt to implement desired levels of privacy by using behavioural mechanisms such as verbal behaviour, nonverbal means, environmental behaviours (e.g. personal space and territory), and culturally defined norms and practices. Verbal privacy mechanisms can be considered from two perspectives, i.e. that of content and structure. Verbal content refers to the substance of verbal communication or "what" is said. Structural aspects of verbal behaviour include what have been termed paraverbal, paralinguistic or linguistic features of speech ("how" it is said). Nonverbal behaviour involves the use of various parts of the body to communicate. It is important to understand these behavioural mechanisms if one is to support the privacy of another person. Environmental privacy mechanisms could be analysed by looking at those who are very close to the person and those who are farther away. Altman (1975), for example, differentiates between clothing and adornment and personal space.

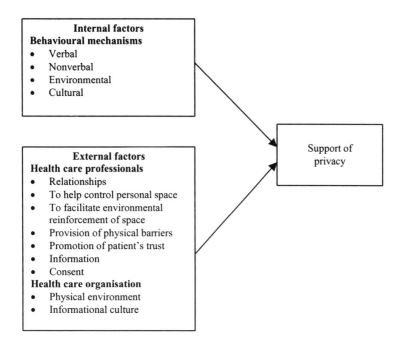

**Figure 6.** Factors supporting privacy

Externally, the most important supporting factors are social relationships and the physical environment. As far as social relationships are concerned, nurses and other health care professionals have the main role in hospital organisations. When people enter public institutions, they are often explicitly obliged to surrender some degree of their privacy. In an institutional setting health professionals may be more anxious about privacy and confidentiality than patients are. Nevertheless, professionals cannot ignore the need of individuals for privacy, and they have a primary moral duty to protect the rights of patients entrusted to their care (Thompson et al. 1994). This duty makes the patient-nurse relationship one of the supporting factors.

In the nursing literature, Meisenheimer (1982) has analysed the concept of personal space and its relevance to nursing practice. She concludes that health care personnel should allow the client to direct the use of his or her personal space. A nurse can allow patients control over their personal space by such simple courtesies as asking permission to enter the client's room or to administer a treatment. Providing explanations before all procedures and not tampering with the objects in the patient's personal space without permission are actions which maintain the patient's domain over his or her private space. Nursing interventions to maintain personal space will 1) help the patient demonstrate control of his or her personal space, 2) facilitate environmental reinforcement of the patient's personal space, 3) provide physical barriers to protect the patient's personal space when treatment necessitates close contact and 4) promote the patient's trust in his or her caretakers.

Physical environment can support privacy, especially when privacy is connected with the concept of territoriality. There is very limited research in the area of physical environment and patient care in hospitals and health care organisations, particularly as far as nursing is concerned. However, Williams (1988) wrote a detailed literature review based on nursing journals and doctoral dissertations. She concluded the review by emphasising the importance of the physical environment, particularly in the care of certain vulnerable populations (e.g. elderly in long-term institutions).

### 3.2 Factors restricting privacy

Privacy can be lost and it is an object of exchange (Schwartz 1968, Laufer & Wolfe 1977). There are two ways people can lose their privacy (Gross 1971): it may be given up (internal), or it may taken away (external, Figure 7). The abandonment of privacy is an inoffensive loss, while deprivation by others is an offensive loss. A person's privacy (or loss of privacy) should not be confused with that person's sense of privacy (or sense of loss of privacy). A person may have privacy while wrongly believing that someone is eavesdropping, and a person may unknowingly have lost some measure of privacy when someone discovers a medical history or chart and discloses its contents to others. What counts as a loss of privacy and what affects an individual's sense of loss of privacy can also vary from society to society and individual to individual, in part because no particular item is intrinsically private (Beauchamp & Childress 1994). Also, a person can have privacy without having control over access by others. At early ages children, for example, have little or no choice of privacy situations (Laufer & Wolfe 1977).

Invasion of privacy is divided into four types (Aiken & Catalano 1994), all described as external ones. Firstly, intrusion upon the seclusion or private concerns of another. This consists of intentional interference with another's interest in solitude or seclusion, regarding his or her personal or private affairs. Eavesdropping upon private conversations, peering into windows, making unwanted telephone calls, illegally searching shopping bags, or invading a person's home are examples. Listening in on hospital telephone calls or searching through a patient's belongings without authorisation may also be considered an invasion of the patients' privacy. In addition, filming or otherwise documenting medical activities without the patient's permission may also be considered an invasion of privacy if it is done for purposes other than treatment of the patient. Secondly, public disclosure of private facts amounts to invasion of privacy. Finally, the two forms of invasion are publicity that places the person in a false light in the public eye, and appropriation of a person's name or likeness.

The regulation of personal information is one of the areas that has been extensively described (Wolfe 1978). In a more community-oriented approach, information regulation has been almost the only perspective on privacy. There are various codes, norms and laws especially for controlling the regulation of personal information and for supporting the privacy of personal information. However, the privacy of personal information has received far less attention in research. Other informational problems include the large proportion of sensitive data in computer systems, and the multitude of users (including physicians, nurses, ward secretaries, administration clerks, medical technicians, and insurance officers) with different information needs and access rights (Ziporyn 1984).

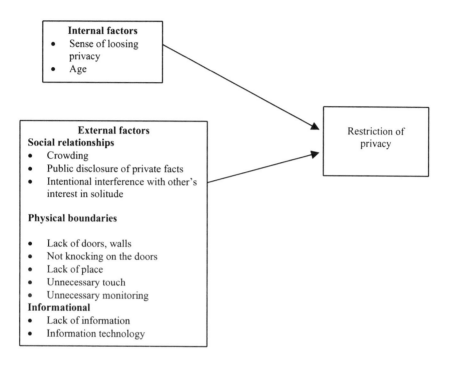

**Figure 7 .** Factors restricting privacy

The moral concern for privacy requires constant vigilance against unnecessary monitoring, examining and questioning of clients. Although they are ultimately intended in the client's best interest, we have seen how they can undermine his or her most fundamental welfare, namely, his or her standing as a person (Muyskens 1982).

Physical boundaries can be seen as a restricting factor. Schwartz (1968) refers to doors and walls and the rules that can open them. He makes a distinction between different types of doors, all of which nonetheless serve to protect privacy. In some studies on privacy in hospital, knocking on the patient's door has been seen as a symbol of disturbing privacy (e.g. Bauer 1994). However, Schwartz (1968) demonstrates very clearly that privacy is not dependent on the availability of lockable doors.

Lack of physical space also has a restrictive effect on privacy. When space becomes scarce, the individual's behaviour is constricted. Reactions to encroachments may take the form of aggressive defence, barrier erection, or communal isolation (Tate 1980). Also, intrusion into any patient's personal space may result in angry behaviour, refusal of procedures or silence (Louis 1981) or produce behavioural deterioration (Nelson & Paluck 1980). Insufficient privacy caused by overcrowded conditions may lead to an increase in social and physical illness, sexual disturbances and aggression (Boucher 1971).

Unnecessary physical touch can also be a factor restricting privacy (Routasalo 1997, Edwards 1998). Nursing has been described as a touching profession (Barnett 1972) and there are quite a few studies into physical touching as part of nursing activities. There can be also a financial link. Justin (1989) says that cost containment measures ignore patients' need for privacy.

## 4. Privacy in empirical studies

### 4.1 General

Research into privacy issues in nursing and midwifery is limited, as has recently been pointed out by Burden (1998). Most studies deal with privacy in relation to bathrooms, particularly for the disabled and those in mental hospitals (e.g. Marr & Pirie 1990, Travers et al. 1992). The need for privacy has been rated as high among psychiatric patients (e.g. Schultz 1977), and it is viewed as extremely important, something to be valued and safeguarded by other patients as well (Schuster 1976a). According to Burden (1998), the drive for most studies in privacy is the need to improve standards of care. Many researchers recommend that in hospital planning privacy should be taken into account (Gainsborough 1970, Tate 1980). Privacy is also connected with nurse staffing levels: privacy can best be guaranteed with higher more staffing levels (Seelye 1982).

Hospital is an environment in which patients have only limited possibilities to control the environment and where they experience losses of privacy (Johnson 1979, see also Annas 1981) and stress (Volicer & Wynne Bohannon 1975, Wilson-Barnett 1979, Davies & Peters 1983). Schuster (1976a) identified four major variables within hospitals, which strongly influence the ability of patients to control or protect their boundaries. These variables are mobility, level of consciousness and awareness, the specific character of patient-to-patient relationships and perception of role. Mobility is the general term depicting the ease with which the patient can move about physically, performing tasks for himself. The substantive level of consciousness and awareness, then, influences the ability to adjust the boundary and allow entry. The specific character of patient-to-patient relationships is the singular situation inside hospitals in which patients share the feeling "we're all in this thing together". Perception of role refers, in part, to the view the individual has of himself as a patient. This also includes his relationships with others in their respective roles.

Patients' territory usually consists of the room (Lane 1989, 1990, Hovi 1990) but they often have to share it with others; it is also the place of work for nurses and other health care professionals. Studies of patients in hospitals or institutions (e.g. Sommer 1969, Hines 1985, Hovi 1990) have reported that patients want to mark their territory in some way, or they select the same place or chair in the room. That is why in elderly nursing care personal belongings have been seen as important for patients' well-being in long-term organisations (McCracken 1987, Calkins 1995, Vaininen et al. 1999).

Physically the hospital environment has many specialities. Design of the rooms and wards, sound-level, colours, light, temperature, weather and other people are different than in most homes. In the nursing literature, Nightingale (1980, first edition 1859) was the first to emphasise the importance of physical environment, having an enormous influence on hospital architecture throughout the world (Thompson & Goldin 1975). More recently, the components of physical environment have been under closer examination. For example, studies into sound levels in hospitals (Falk & Woods 1973, Woods & Falk 1974, Ogilvie 1980, Davies and Peters 1983, Keefe 1984, see also the review by Williams 1988) suggest that problems are caused to patients and most of them recommend that the noise level should be reduced. Some studies make a distinction between sound from mechanical sources and from discussions between other patients and staff. Haslam (1970) found that patients were more disturbed by conversations than by sound from mechanical sources. In the study by Hilton (1976) on the effects of sound on sleep, sounds created by staff were most frequently the disturbing factor.

In Davies and Peters' (1983) study, the hospital itself was seen as a source of stress to patients. A total of 25 patients and their nurses were interviewed. The patients were interviewed twice, after about one week and three weeks in hospital. Both groups agreed that the stress items derived from the hospital environment and routines, such as noise, privacy, early morning routines and toileting. The most stressful factors were thinking about home, not having visitors, early morning routines and noise on the ward. Privacy was not among the most stressful factors, and nurses considered it more stressful than the patients. Toileting and using commode were among the more stressful factors, but not at the top of the list.

The physical environment can also cause problems for the fulfilment of patients' basic needs. For example, Travers et al. (1992) investigated the hospital toilet facilities in 13 wards in a large provincial teaching hospital in the United Kingdom. According to the results none of the toilets (n = 17) met the standards recommended by the British Standards Institution. The worst facilities were found on a ward accommodating elderly patients, where the toilets were unsuitable for use by disabled people and bedside commodes had to be used instead. The authors conclude that it is unlikely that the hospital under investigation is alone in its inadequate toilet facilities and refer to the study carried out in Edinburgh, Scotland (Sklaroff & Atkinson 1987).

Teaching hospitals represent a special case as far as privacy is concerned. According to Beauchamp and Childress (1994) only very few patients understand the extent of their potential loss of privacy when they enter a teaching hospital, where professionals in training often seek access to them for reasons that have nothing to do with their care. Relevant information about teaching hospitals therefore should be disclosed to the patient as part of the consent process on admission, and patients should also have the right to limit access of professionals and students not involved in their care (see also Cantrell 1978).

Patients' privacy is also an important issue in research ethics, especially in clinical experiments (Cooper 1991). It includes the implementation of ethical rules during the whole research process, but especially limiting the use of personal information to the purposes for which it was collected and preventing the disclosure of personal information outside the research team.

Information is very important for patients in hospital (e.g. Leino-Kilpi et al. 1993). In the study by Volicer and Wynne Bohannon (1975), the most stressful factors listed by 261 hospital patients included not being told the diagnosis, not knowing for sure what illness one had, not knowing the results or reasons for one's treatments and not having one's questions answered by the staff. Lind et al. (1989) also emphasised that communication about various aspects of the disease is a central issue for patients.

Data integrity, protection and preventing inaccuracies is one of the basic areas of privacy protection in hospital (Callens 1993, Smith 1996). This is particularly important today with the continuing growth and development of modern technology. The research evidence suggests that the meaning of technology to privacy varies. Some authors say that technology is a risk or danger for privacy (Hiller 1981, Milholland 1994, Brannigan & Beier 1995, Hoge 1995, Chou 1996), or more specifically computerised databases (Rittman & Gorman 1992), computer-based record-keeping (Milholland 1994) and telemedicine (e.g. Brannigan & Beier 1995, Crowe & McDonald 1997, Guttman-McGabe 1997, Eliasson & Poropatich 1998). Problems have also been identified in certain special areas such as dental care (Szekely et al. 1996). However, not all agree: in a study by Gardner & Lundsgaarde (1994, see also Dierks 1993), technology was found to have no influence on privacy.

Questions of informational privacy are also relevant in medication, pharmacy services inside and outside the hospital and laboratory examinations. Schommer & Wiederholt (1995, see also Beardsley et al. 1977, Kelly et al. 1990) identified different variables that affect pharmacist-patient communication. Privacy was one of the variables tested and was connected mainly with the information given to patients. Allison et al. (1994) studied the screening services for risk factors for coronary heart disease in retail pharmacies in UK. One problem for pharmacists was the lack of space available to ensure patient privacy and confidentiality during screening. Raisch (1993) surveyed pharmacists to evaluate their perceptions of barriers to performing cognitive services in community pharmacy. One of the perceived barriers to counselling patients was lack of privacy.

In laboratory examinations, problems of privacy can be encountered in examinations of HIV or AIDS patients (e.g. Chipeur 1993, Dickenson 1994). Leino-Kilpi et al. (1997), however, investigated the realisation of patients' rights (n = 203) in the most common types of laboratory examinations using a questionnaire. One area of rights was privacy. The results suggested that privacy protection was realised reasonably well. Laboratory staff did not disclose the results of examinations to relatives or friends without the patient's permission; the patient's name and social security code was not mentioned within the hearing of other patients; staff did not speak about the examinations within hearing of other patients; and the results remained confidential within the hospital organisation. Some patients, however, had their suspicions about the computerised system: only 30 % believed that their data was safe in the hospital's computer system.

In the context of professional relationships, privacy can be seen as part of confidentiality (Parrott et al. 1989). In the study by Parrott et al. (1989), there were three groups of subjects (N = 427). The majority (N = 318) were solicited from workplaces and an apartment complex; the second group (n = 43) were students and the final group (n = 66) were individuals participating in another study. The subjects ranged in age from 16 to 77, with a mean of 27. All the participants had been to see a medical doctor within the past six months. A 10-item questionnaire was used. The results showed that 34 % the of respondents agreed or strongly agreed that having to undress before a physician was a violation of their privacy. Almost half or 48 % considered undressing with a nurse present to be invasive; and 55 % considered undressing parts of the body unrelated to the reason for a medical visit to be a violation. One-fourth (25 %) considered recommendations to join a support group invasive, and 28 % viewed questions about the use of leisure time as violations. In terms of issues more psychological in nature, 54 % of the respondents considered reference to morality to be an assault of privacy; 40 % considered being told they are irresponsible about taking care of their health to be invasive; 22 % considered the issue of being asked to participate in medical research to be a violation of privacy; and 48 % considered the question about how many people they have had sex with in the past six months to be a violation.

Referring to stress in hospital (Volicer & Wynne Bohannon 1975), the social dimension of having strangers sleep in the same room does not seem to be very stressful for patients; also having to eat at different times than you usually do does not stress the patients. By contrast, not getting pain medication when it was needed or being fed through tubes were quite considerable sources of stress.

Experiences of privacy seem to be partly connected with the respondents' background. For example, in the study by Parrot et al. (1989) in USA females perceived more violations than males; this was particularly clear in the case of undressing. Younger patients found that the situation where a patient must undress before a doctor to be more invasive than older persons did. The authors conclude young women in particular are at risk of privacy violation. The issue of privacy encompasses not only publicly discussed assaults on individuals' privacy, such as information collection and dissemination, but also personal concerns. What must be regarded as part of patients' privacy is not only how physicians handle patients' private files, but how physicians facilitate patients' perceptions of physical, interactional and psychological privacy.

Patients and professionals may differ in their views on privacy. For example, Bäck & Wikblad (1998) explored patients' (n = 120) and nurses' (n = 42) attitudes towards privacy and whether nurses' perceptions of patients' privacy needs corresponded with the patients' own reported needs. The findings indicated that nurses mostly estimated the patient's needs for privacy as higher than the patient's own rating. Being able to talk to the physician in private was given the highest preference. Patients in long-term care had higher privacy preferences than those in acute care. Younger patients showed a tendency towards higher privacy preferences, especially on the preference to be allowed to talk to the physician in private. In addition, patients with a higher level of education showed a tendency towards overall higher privacy preferences compared with patients with less education. Patients who had their first hospital experience showed a tendency towards lower ratings on most items than did those who had been hospitalised before, while females had higher overall scores for privacy than males, and younger patients had higher privacy preferences compared with older patients.

## 4.2 Privacy and care of the elderly and chronically ill

The subject of privacy and elderly people, especially those in nursing homes, has received considerable attention in nursing research as well as in certain other disciplines. In nursing homes and long-term facilities, nurses seem to know what is best for their clients, but there is a lack of time and resources (Armstrong-Esther et al. 1989, 1994) and the activities and procedures are performed in a routine manner (Liukkonen 1990, Waters 1994). Nurses may also assess patients' privacy needs stereotypically (Farrell 1991). This lack can also have an impact on the realisation of privacy.

Studies in the area of elderly care are focused in six:

> ➤ Importance and definitions of privacy
> ➤ Personal space and territoriality
> ➤ Physical environment
> ➤ Information
> ➤ Cultural issues

### Importance and definitions of privacy

Privacy has been described as important to elderly in institutions (e.g. Johnson 1979, Louis 1981, Mattiasson & Hemberg 1998). Mattiasson and Hemberg (1998) say that intimacy and privacy are closely connected with each other. With increasing age elderly patients continue to need more and more help with actions that used to belong to a very personal sphere. On the other hand, elderly patients have a need for respect for their privacy, a rightful wish not to be forced into more intimacy than the care situation and care actions demand. Confused patients in particular should be taken into account. Some studies (e.g. Armstrong-Esther et al. 1989) indicate that nurses tend to contact the confused patients less often than those who are oriented.

There are some studies that have looked at how elderly people define the concept of privacy. Roosa (1982) questioned residents about their understanding of privacy. Solitude was the most frequently chosen definition of privacy, with self-evaluation identified as its most appreciated function. Violations of residents' sense of privacy occurred mainly in connection with hygiene and elimination, but also when too many roommates had to share sleeping quarters or the architectural design made it impossible to spend time alone (Raphael 1979, Willcocks et al. 1987). The patient's sense of dignity and privacy is still violated. It seems still to be common practice that residents have to use a commode in front of their roommates (Bauer 1994).

*Personal space and territoriality*

The main research interest has been with personal space (e.g. Gioiella 1978, Phillips 1979, Louis 1981) and territoriality, even though (as Louis 1981 observes) there is a lack of empirical research into personal space among people over age 65. In the future there will apparently be a need for more research in this area as well, mainly because of the growing number of elderly people (e.g. WHO 1997).

In some of these studies (e.g. Gioiella 1978) age is identified as the most important predictor of preferred personal space, which contradicts other findings (e.g. Johnson 1979, Geden & Begeman 1981) that age made no significant difference at all. Louis (1981) studied 40 (= n) residents (65 - 90 years) in an apartment housing unit for the elderly in the United States. The purpose was to identify a baseline for personal space of independently functioning elderly people. On the basis of the results, personal space needs are not the same for all people. Residents should be approached slowly and one should obtain at least implied consent to come closer if the professional must to do that. In this context, personal space needs were greater laterally than anteriorly, which contradicts common theories that a person is more sensitive to a face-to-face intrusion. In Johnson's study (1979, see also Allekian 1973), the lowest level of anxiety was reported during intrusions caused by nurses when they sat on beds or entered the room without knocking; higher levels of anxiety were reported when residents were intruders. Females were significantly more anxious about intrusion than males.

Physical touch can also influence personal space. In Finland, Routasalo (1997) analysed physical touch on three long-term wards with elderly patients using direct observation, interviews and video recordings. She observed touching episodes (182 observed situations, 94 patients and 32 nurses) and interviewed 25 elderly patients and 30 nurses. Patients experienced touching in different ways: it was generally accepted when it was necessary for obtaining help or when it was interpreted as having a positive nature. The author, however, points out that the touch could also be used as a symbol of power and domination by the nurse.

Tate (1980) describes the need for personal space in institutions for the elderly. She says that aggressive behaviour is not uncommon in defence on personal space. Invasion of personal space raises the individual's anxiety level and can provoke aggressive or violent behaviour; individuals differ in their need for space. DeLong (1970) theorises that the elderly require three functionally different spaces in their institutional settings: private, semiprivate/semi-public and public. On the basis of his study it is possible to identify certain spatial-behavioural relationships: for instance, private rooms reduce aggression and increase cooperation among elderly. Studies on resident satisfaction with and desire for private rooms are not conclusive.

The concept of territoriality has also been used in studies of elderly people (Johnson 1978, 1979). Johnson (1978) reported that institutionalised residents who were socially engaged but who had physical limitations were more anxious about territorial intrusions than patients with no physical limitations. In 1979, Johnson collected data from 31 (= n) elderly residents in the United States. Ninety percent of them established territories in their rooms, 52 % exhibited high territorial behaviour, and 6 % had high anxiety towards territorial intrusion. Type of room showed no clear connection with the level of anxiety; females responded with higher anxiety towards territorial intrusion, and previous occupation was also a relevant factor.

Roberto et al. (1997) describe the rights of residents in long-term care facilities in the US. These rights include the right to dignified and respectful treatment, responsiveness to individual needs, consideration of personal interests and being a decision-maker. More specifically, they say, these rights are interpreted or defined as the right to privacy (e.g. knocking before entering residents' room) and choice (e.g. what residents eat or who they spend time with). Residents also have the right to be informed about their medical conditions, and to be free from physical and chemical restraints. In their questionnaire study with 83 certified nursing assistants and 62 nurses in five nursing homes, the authors asked nursing staff about residents' rights. On the basis of the results, nursing staff in long-term care facilities are knowledgeable of resident rights, but the actual implementation of residents' rights in everyday work appears to be a difficult task.

*Physical environment*

The environment of elderly people has also been investigated outside health care organisations. Moos and Lemke (1984) conducted a study in California on the facilities of the elderly, referring to their choice in daily living, participation in facility operation and participation in setting policies. The facilities included in the comparison were skilled nursing facilities, residential care facilities and apartment facilities. They found considerable variability in the opportunities for choice and control available in these settings: the skilled nursing facilities did not allow so much choice and control than the others. The authors suggest more alternatives in the housing of the elderly population.

Faletti (1984) has analysed the functional ability of elderly people from the point of view of the person environment problem. The extension of independence and autonomy for older persons in community settings has been a major concern for researchers and practitioners in ageing. Faletti divided the literature into two parts: the first has concentrated on the development of person environment models of adaptive behaviour in the elderly, the second has sought to reflect the person-environment perspective in the design of housing and environment for older persons. He describes a conceptual model relating to task performance and environment demand, including the border for autonomy.

Several authors have described ward experiences and recommended practical improvements in nursing homes by reference to privacy (Trierweiler 1978, Johnson 1979, Tate 1980, Elliott 1982, Davis 1984, Vousden 1987, Bauer 1994). Tate (1980) has proposed a model of behaviour resulting from inadequate personal space. A special focus in this model is on the environment for institutionalised elderly, and Tate has various suggestions for improving physical environments. These suggestions include the limitation of the size of the nursing homes and number of residents, provision of private rooms and private bathrooms, limitation of the size of public areas (such as sitting rooms), teaching the staff to honour the privacy of patients and furniture arrangements (see also Trierweiler 1978) to maximise feelings of security and privacy.

The meal situation in geriatric care has been studied by Sidenvall et al. (1994) and Davies and Snaith (1980). In the study by Sidenvall et al. (1994), the ethnographic method was employed to study 18 mentally oriented patients. Most of the patients were satisfied with the menu. They were classified into three groups according to the effects of their motor dysfunctions on eating competence, their personal standards of table manners, and their contact with others: those with severe eating problems, moderate eating problems and eating with ease. The nurses enrolled saw the dining room as their workplace and their measures as part of the routine. This, according to the authors, led to problems in nursing care. With respect to privacy, elderly patients suffered because of their own limited eating competence and the experience of other patients' problems.

In Finnish nursing home, Palohuhta (1995) investigated the views of long-term patients' relatives (n = 15) of the physical hospital environment. The physical environment was limited in the health centre concerned, mainly because of the patient's health conditions. Hygiene and physical needs were adequately met, but relatives complained that nurses were under too much time pressure and that staffing levels were inadequate. This made it impossible to meet patients' spiritual and social needs. The rooms were small and provided no stimuli. The toilets and bathrooms offered no independence to patients.

Ryhänen and Vaittinen (1994) interviewed 40 patients (over 65 years) in nursing homes and health centres. On the basis of their results, the elderly people were quite satisfied with their physical environment. The main problems were lack of toilets, cold toilets and bathrooms and restlessness and noise in patient rooms. It was impossible for patients in rooms with many others to have any personal territory of their own. Freedom, safety, peace and privacy were their main concerns.

*Information*

Information is also important for elderly people, and lack of privacy has been reported to be a problem in situations related to patient information (Athlin et al. 1992, Bouchard 1993). It is not uncommon for patients to receive information about their diagnosis and surgery in front of other patients on the ward (Bouchard 1993).

*Cultural issues*

Privacy can be experienced differently in different countries and cultural areas. For example, there is an interesting comparison between Sweden and the UK (Barron 1990) about privacy. Data were collected by participant observation, interviews and questionnaires amongst patients (n = 80), nurses (n = 76) and relatives (n = 61). There seems to be a difference between these two countries in the nursing context: British nurses were more "practically" based, while replies from Swedish nurses were almost totally based on matters of principle. The nurses were asked how would they maintain patients' privacy. In Britain, the most common response was "Drawing curtains round the bed while patient is washing or dressing". In Sweden, the most common answer was, to treat patient as an individual. Some results based on patient and relative data reveal problems of privacy in both the countries: the door to the toilet was not always closed, curtains were not used, nurses did not knock on the room or toilet door, and nurses failed to maintain the dignity of patients when they help them with washing. Privacy, however, was very important to all groups of respondents.

### 4.3 Privacy and acute care

It seems that there has been less research into questions of privacy in acute care settings than in long-term institutions (Bauer 1994). There are, however, anecdotal articles which emphasise the importance of privacy in emergency departments (Johnston 1988), in the search for patient identification in emergencies (George & Quattrone 1985), in recovery rooms (Minckley 1968), and with critically ill patients (Roberts 1986).

The physical dimension of privacy is also clearly to be seen in acute care. There are only a few studies, most of them from the US, but one also from Germany (Bauer 1994). Minckley's study (1968) is one of the first in the nursing literature. She examined the need for personal space among more than 600 recovery room clients. She labelled the phenomenon she observed as civil inattention, the attempt between strangers to avoid one another's presence while forced to be physically close. Minckley concludes that such close proximity is clearly an uncomfortable situation for patients, yet a necessity in immediate postoperative circumstances. The specific behaviours noted were: failure to recognise adjacent patients, although nurses were readily identified at a distance; closed eyes, heads under covers or turned towards the walls; and much verbalised anxiety to return to one's room.

In the 1970s Allekian (1973, 1974) researched intrusions into territory and personal space and anxiety-producing factors among patients in the US. She interviewed 76 adults. According to the results of these studies, the entry of a nurse into the room without knocking was responded to with indifference, whereas someone looking through one's belongings, or removal of one's bedside table, or opening/closing one's windows or shades, all without permission, provoked strong reactions. Personal space intrusions did not seem to be as anxiety-producing as one might have assumed. Intrusions into one's territory, however, created strong annoyance. Santa-Maria (1982) later used the modified version of Allekian's questionnaire and studied 584 patients in Philippine hospitals and found differences between certain patients groups. Lane (1989) also used Allekian's questionnaire with 80 patients and 80 nurses. On the basis of these results, nurses expected male patients to have more negative experiences than female patients when personal space and territory was violated. Among patients, however, the results were precisely the opposite (see also Parrott et al. 1989).

Problems of privacy have been identified among cancer patients receiving chemotherapy on an outpatient basis. Repeated visits require a continuous commitment on the part of patients as well as dependence on the clinic. Thus, for the majority of patients, the physical environment of the outpatient clinic will be part of their lives for long periods of time. Bouchard (1993) conducted a survey in Canada with 55 outpatients ranging from 38 to 78 years of age (mean 56 years). Forty-six of the patients were female, and 43 English-speaking. Concerned primarily with the physical environment, this study focused on the aspects of physical comfort, privacy, social interaction, safety, and information and counselling. The patients identified two aspects as a problem: lack of privacy and confidentiality of information and discomfort associated with odours. The majority were satisfied with those environmental aspects that encouraged social interaction and provided physical comfort and counselling.

In the study by Bouchard (1993) 22 patients (n = 55) were dissatisfied with the privacy provided in the waiting room and the treatment rooms. Lack of privacy was a primary concern of patients who were fatigued, nauseated, or felt ill. Thirty one patients expressed dissatisfaction with the confidentiality of information. The main concern appeared to be the staff's verbal disclosure of information regarding their medical situation in public areas of the clinic; and 24 patients complained about unpleasant odours in the waiting room (e.g. cleaning liquids, coffee). Seeing other patients who had lost weight and looked ill, seeing patients who had lost their hair, or hearing other patients talk about the side-effects of treatment, all made patients worry about what would happen to themselves (Nicholas 1988). Morning rounds in the hospital have a special role in the realisation of privacy, at least among cancer patients (Blanchard et al. 1986).

The social dimension of privacy can be identified in the study by Geden and Begeman (1981), who compared personal space preferences of 60 hospitalised adults in hospital and home settings and compared whether these patients assigned different personal space to a family member, a nurse, a physician, or a stranger. The physician was placed as close as family members, whereas the nurse was located significantly further away, the stranger furthest; Stratton (1981), however, found no difference between nurse and physician. Schuster's (1976a,b) model of interpersonal distancing within hospitalisation was based on the meaning of privacy for patients. However, as Bauer (1994) has observed, this model is difficult to follow.

In Finland, Jantunen et al. (1994) carried out a questionnaire study with patients (n = 135) on medical wards, hospitalised because of infectious diseases. The age of the respondents varied between 15 to 84, mean 48 years. Both men and women were included in the sample, mostly educated at the comprehensive school level. The patients were asked to define the meaning of privacy: for 44 % it meant having control over personal information, for 32 % territoriality, and for 15 % self-determination; 9 % had other, mixed definitions. For 45 % privacy in hospital was very important, and only for 3 % not at all important. Confidentiality of personal information was even more important: 66 % described it as very important. During their hospital stay, however, 21 % of the patients said that their privacy had been poorly taken into account; 18 % had no opinion, 47 % said it had been taken into account well and 14 % very well. The most problematic aspect as far as privacy was concerned was the patients' need for help with personal hygiene (about 40 %) and elimination (about 50 %). The patients usually used withdrawal (60 %) as a means for privacy. One-fifth of the respondents thought that staff always knocked on the door, while 16 % said never and 22 % very rarely. The authors have a number of concrete suggestions for developing privacy in hospital settings. One of the more general proposals says that much can be done to improve patient privacy without any financial investment, i.e. by intervening in the behaviour of nurses and planning of care.

In Germany, Bauer (1994) carried out a study on privacy in acute care hospitals. Using patient interviews (n = 20) in the first phase as well as questionnaires and the rank-ordering technique, she created a theory of patients' privacy in hospitals. The study was conducted in a 502-bed acute care hospital with a large rural catchment area in Germany;

the hospital was also a teaching hospital. The categories listed in Table 5 demonstrate patients' concerns about their privacy in an acute care setting (Bauer 1994):

**Table 5.** Categories of privacy in acute care setting

**Categories of privacy**

Privacy in general
Privacy in the hospital in contrast to the home
Fear of exposure of personal identity
Personal autonomy
Fear of physical exposure of body
Territoriality
Personal space
Intimate distance
Effect of invasion of privacy on the individual
The individual as part of a patient community
Coping mechanisms/reactions to invasion of privacy
Features of the hospital experience that should be changed

The category of "Fear of physical exposure of body" included such areas as washing facilities, focus on the treatment of intimate areas of the body, elimination and entering the room. Some of the patients were worried about the level of hygiene in hospital and about the cleanliness of washing facilities. Being washed seems to mean different things to different patients: for instance, some patients are uncomfortable with being washed by a stranger, or by a person of the opposite sex. It seems to be extremely embarrassing to use a bedpan or commode. It is also embarrassing to expose the contents of drainage bags. For some of the patients, screens were not at all necessary; for some they were essential and for some they were essential for examinations or dressing. Opening the doors without warning does not disturb some of the patients, but some thought that the possibility of the door being opened is dreadful.

For most of the interviewed patients, their territory consisted of the bed and bedside table, but also wardrobe, toilet places, and the whole room were mentioned. Territory in surgical wards was also the topic in the Finnish study by Hovi (1990), who interviewed 30 surgical patients. Most of them also mentioned the bed plus the table as their own territory, and only very few thought that any area outside of the room could be their territory. Within one's territory there should be reasonable safety of belongings and enough place for personal belongings. In the study by Edwards (1998) on an acute medical ward, personal space was the area within the curtain, for example bed, chair and locker; this study was based on interviews with six patients and seven nurses on one ward in the UK.

In Bauer's (1994) questionnaire study the data were collected from the same wards where the interviews were carried out; 117 males and 83 females took part in the study. The questionnaire comprised most of the same areas as the categories based on the interviews. The informational dimension of privacy is clearly in evidence in the category of "Fear of exposure of personal identity" (12 items). Most patients agreed, for example, that personal matters should not be discussed in front of others, they did not want to have talk about private matters in front of others, they had difficulties being in private with visitors and they thought that telephone calls attract the attention of all other patients in the room.

In the category of "Personal autonomy" (5 items, Bauer 1994), most of the patients thought that privacy in hospital is limited because one has to fit into a system and obey the rules. In the category of "Fear of physical exposure" (20 items), most patients were of the opinion that they would try anything to avoid using a bedpan/commode and that one of the most dreadful things would be to use the commode in front of others; they make no distinction between male and female nurses assisting them in personal activities, they try to get a room with en suite facilities and smell and noise are even more embarrassing than being watched sitting on a bedpan/commode. In the category of "Territoriality" (9 items) the patients described their views on things in the room and the size of the room: most of them did not want to get an additional bed in their room, they thought that the more patients in the room, the less privacy there is, they did not wanted the nurse to open their bedside locker or wardrobe without permission, and they did not want to have a larger than a two-bed room. In the category of "Personal space" (2 items), the patients said they did not want the beds to be too close and they needed quite a bit of space around them. In the category of "Effect of invasion of privacy on individual" (4 items), most patients were of the opinion that if there is a good relationship between patients, it does not matter very much if one's privacy is invaded. There were differences between genders and age-groups in each of the categories. The authors concludes that the results tended to support the interview findings.

In the third, rank-ordering part of Bauer's (1994) study, all groups of patients rated the use of a bedpan/commode and the treatment of intimate areas as the worst privacy-intruding events, while other events such as entering the room without knocking (also Johnson 1979) and being recognised as a hospitalised patient, were judged as relatively tolerable. Based on all three parts of the study, Bauer (1994) made a preliminary model of reaction and outcome of privacy invasion depending on the individual's constitution. Its most important feature is that individuals with a high need of privacy who are prevented from employing appropriate measures to maintain their desired level of privacy suffer from stress. This model, however, should be tested in future research.

## 4.4 Privacy in gynaecological and maternity care

Research into privacy issues in midwifery practice and maternity care is limited, as Burden (1998) points out. More generally speaking, ethical issues and dilemmas faced by midwives have also received relatively little coverage in the ethical literature (Frith 1998a), even thought there are quite many clinically oriented studies (Lydon-Rochelle & Albers 1993). In midwifery, however, as Burden (1998) states, there is a pressing need for example in the United Kingdom to address questions relating to the impact of the care environment if the objective of women-centred care is to be achieved (see Intimate examinations 1997, Barclay 1998, Frith 1998a). This section looks at studies in maternity care within the hospital organisation and also at some related topics, such as patients in gynaecological examinations.

The physical dimension of privacy is also present in research into maternity care. One of the focal areas of research has been the delivery room as a physical environment (Carey & Helander 1993), the importance of which has also been emphasised in textbooks (Balaskas & Gordon 1989, Bobak et al. 1989). In Finland, Carey and Helander (1993) studied the self-determination of mothers (n = 475) and the links between the physical environment of the delivery-room and the realisation of self-determination. Mothers expected to deliver in a cosy, but technologically safe environment. Most of them (94 %) were satisfied with the delivery-rooms and 93 % felt that the physical environment has an impact on the success of childbirth. Unpleasant feelings during the delivery process included having shaving, various gynaecological examinations and pain. Some mothers referred to the radio being too loud, sounds from other rooms as well as lack of space in delivery rooms.

In a maternity ward environment, Burden (1998) conducted a study in the UK on the use of curtain positioning strategies as a means of achieving and maintaining privacy. This study employed an ethnographic approach. The subjects under study were women within the ward, excluding those on their first day following Caesarean section, and comprised both mothers and infants. Documentary evidence (midwifery notes and care charts) and participant observation were used for data collection. Based on the data, the strategies employed by women on the ward included complete closure for total withdrawal, semi-closure for seeking information or support and partial closure of curtains around the individual's bed space for periods of solitude or rest. Complete closure signalled the need for total withdrawal and reserve, women physically introduced barriers to maintain their privacy. Complete closure can be classified into two elements, either short (5-10 minutes) or prolonged. Semi-closure of ward curtains is a strategy adopted by women who either require support from other women, or staff, during the antenatal period, or is used by women in their postnatal period to gain solitude. Observations of the rooms which contained only antenatal women showed that these women introduced semi-closure of curtains in order to attract the attention of the professionals as a means of information gathering. In the postnatal wards (or mixed antenatal and postnatal wards), the curtains were closed especially for breastfeeding. Also, the mothers did not feel confident in handling their babies and they wanted not to be seen to be performing inadequately. Partial closure of the curtains was a strategy adopted by most women throughout the day. Women usually required periods of solitude either to try to sleep or to read. The author emphasises that midwives should be aware of this form of non-verbal communication and act appropriately. She also suggests comparative studies within general wards where men and women are mixed or where clients are confined to bed.

Gynaecological examinations are in a very intimate area and, according to Barclay (1998) each year the General Medical Council in the UK receives complaints from patients who feel that doctors behaved improperly or roughly during an intimate examination. In Intimate examinations (1997), a report prepared by the working party of the Royal College of Obstetricians and Gynaecologists, there are recommendations relating to dignity, modesty and sensitivity. For example, intimate examinations should be conducted in a private room, women should be allowed to undress privately, unnecessary nudity should be avoided and the examinations should be justifiable. In Finland, a study by Niemi (1994, see also Emerson 1973) showed that examinations of genitals and undressing were unpleasant to urological male and female patients. In the qualitative study by Edwards (1998) about space and touch, there seemed to be some differences between men and women: female patients remarked that they preferred female nurses for intimate tasks (such as bathing and toileting purposes). Emerson (1973), in his interesting analysis, describes the differences of the reality of patients and professionals in gynaecological examinations: understanding the patient's reality provides the basis for successful examinations.

Information is also important for pregnant mothers, during delivery and in postnatal care (e.g. Frith 1998a). The informational dimension of privacy is present, for example, when artificial reproductive technologies are used (Frith 1998 b).

There are certain special interventions or examinations during pregnancy, delivery and the postnatal period which involve an obvious risk of privacy being infringed upon. For example, Kruse (1984) studied women's reactions to electronic fetal monitoring during labour by mailing a questionnaire to a random sample of 110 women two to five months postpartum. Of the 75 women who responded and in whom the fetal monitor had been used, 74 gave an overall positive response to fetal monitoring and it was not seen as an invasion of privacy.

# Informed consent in the literature

## 1. General

A database search was carried out on Medline express using the keywords "informed consent" and "patient informed consent". Between 1965 and 1998, a total of 10,621 abstracts have been published on related subjects. The search with the keyword "patient informed consent" produced 56 abstracts. Manual analysis of the abstracts and publications revealed a greater number of empirical studies in this field.

The ethical doctrine of informed consent is derived from respect for the patient's autonomy, as well as the patient's vulnerability (Segest 1995). Today, informed consent is a central concept in modern medical and nursing ethics (Broggi 1995). Historically, the roots of informed consent can be traced back to the Enlightenment ideals of humanism, liberalism and to human rights thinking. This tradition was grounded in the view that the human individual has certain inalienable rights that must be guaranteed to all people in all circumstances (Lindqvist 1980).

The concept of informed consent was first applied to medical experimentation during the 1947 Nuremberg Trials (Dyer & Bloch 1987). Ever since the horrifying accounts of medical experiments in concentration camps presented at these trials, the issue of consent has been at the forefront of biomedical ethics (Beauchamp & Childress 1994). Therefore, the doctrine of informed consent was developed as a legal mechanism for extending the liability of physicians in the event of injury to the patient (Kaufman 1983).

In the United States and elsewhere the judicial system began to apply the principle of informed consent to resolving individual cases relating to medical care and treatment, thus endorsing it juridically. Interest groups formed by private citizens, for their part, began to advocate patient rights to access information and to take an active part in decisions concerning their own care and treatment (Lindqvist 1980). Questions of informed consent were primarily discussed in relation to surgery: in order to conduct an operation, the patient was required to consent (Dyer & Bloch 1987).

Informed consent promotes self-determinism, rational decision-making in an area that is of vital concern to the individual (Sriram et al. 1989). Ideally, the doctrine contemplates mutual participation between the patient and doctor in a process of shared decision-making (President's Commission 1982, 15-39). In nursing, informed consent is a process that occurs through the course of the nurse-patient relationship, assumes the ethical imperative of giving patients comprehensive information, allowing them to make independence choices (Davis 1988, Scanlon & Fleming 1989, Selekman 1989, Barnes et al. 1998). During this process explicit communication of information is provided that would be relevant for a patient or experimental subject to decide whether or not to have a particular treatment or to participate in a particular experiment (Dyer & Bloch 1987).

In recent years the focus in discussions on informed consent has shifted from the physician's or researcher's obligation to disclose information to the quality of a patient's or subject's understanding and consent. The forces behind this shift of emphasis have been autonomy-driven and primarily external to codes of medical and research ethics (Beauchamp & Childress 1994).

## 2. The concept of informed consent

"Consent" derives from the Latin com- + sentire, i.e. to feel, hence to feel together. It means "agree", "assent", or "give permission" and indicates involvement of the will or feelings and compliance with what is requested or desired. Implicit in the definition is a community of feeling, a shared trust which goes beyond a mere explicit contractual arrangement (Dyer & Bloch 1987).

Discussing the problems surrounding informed consent, Beauchamp and Childress (1994) say that different definitions of informed consent often include descriptions of an obligation to make disclosure rather than a meaning of informed consent. Considerable vagueness also surrounds the term of informed consent, creating a need to shape the concept so that its meaning is more stable and suitable (see Beauchamp & Childress 1994). Further, according to Simón (1995), informed consent is an unavoidable reality within the area of health relations. Therefore, it is necessary to be familiar with the basic elements which constitute an understanding of the concept of informed consent, described as components of informed consent (Dyer & Bloch 1987, Gillett 1989) or analytical components of informed consent (Meisel & Roth 1981). Other authors have used the term "elements of informed consent" (Sprung & Winick 1989, Aiken & Catalano 1994, Beauchamp & Childress 1994). The Table below gives some examples of the different definitions that have been employed (Table 6).

**Table 6.** Definitions of informed consent

| Authors | Examples of definitions |
| --- | --- |
| Meisel & Roth (1981) | Analytical components of informed consent: competence, disclosure, understanding, voluntariness and consent. |
| Dyer & Bloch (1987) | The concept of informed consent has three components: it must be informed, voluntary and competent. |
| Gillett (1989) | Components included in informed consent are accuracy and adequate information; reasoned decision with lack of coercion, followed by a valid consent given. |
| Sprung & Winick (1989) | Elements of informed consent: disclosure of information, competency, understanding, voluntariness and decision-making. |
| Aiken & Catalano (1994) | The elements of informed consent: a patient has been provided with sufficient information to make an intelligent decision to accept or reject treatment based on a full disclosure of the facts. |
| Beauchamp & Childress (1994) | Consent to an intervention is informed if (and perhaps only if) one is competent to act, receives a thorough disclosure, comprehends the disclosure and acts voluntarily. |

Different elements of informed consent: threshold elements (precondition) such as competence (to understand and to decide) and voluntariness (in deciding); information elements such as disclosure (of material information), recommendation (of a plan) and understanding; and consent elements which includes decision (in favour of a plan) and authorisation (of the chosen plan). (Beachamp & Childress 1994.) Further, in order for patients to provide informed consent, they must receive adequate information, they must understand this information and they should consent voluntarily (Schachter et al. 1994, see also Generalitat de Catalunya 1997).

According to the British Medical Association (1995) the three main prerequisites for valid consent are competence, information and voluntariness. These can be further broken down into several fundamental points as prerequisites for informed consent (Table 7).

**Table 7.** Prerequisites for informed consent

**Prerequisites**

- The ability to understand that there is a choice and that choices have consequences;
- A willingness to make a choice (including the choice that someone else chooses the treatment);
- An understanding of the nature and purpose of the proposed procedure;
- An understanding of the proposed procedure's risks and side effects;
- An understanding of the alternatives to the proposed procedure and the risks attached to them; the consequences of no treatment;
- Freedom from pressure.

In general, the role of the doctrine of informed consent is to ensure that what is done is what the patient would himself determine he wants done, having been reasonably and properly informed and having completely voluntarily and understandingly consented (Herbert 1980). According to Beauchamp and Childress (1994), informed consent consists in autonomous authorisation by individuals of a medical intervention or of involvement in research. In the first sense, a person must do more than express agreement or comply with a proposal; he or she must authorise through an act of informed consent and voluntary consent. Therefore, informed consent in the first sense occurs if and only if a patient or subject, with substantial understanding and in substantial absence of control by others, intentionally authorises a professional to do something. In the second sense, informed consent is analysable in terms of the social rules of consent in institutions that must obtain legally valid consent from patients or subjects before proceeding with therapeutic procedures or research. Informed consents are not necessarily autonomous acts under these rules and sometimes are not even meaningful authorisations. It refers only to an institutionally or legally effective authorisation, as determined by prevailing rules.

According to Simón (1995), the question of patient competence is crucial to informed consent because if a patient is considered incompetent or incapable, that patient's right to make decisions concerning him- or herself will be withdrawn. Competence or capacity, when taken to its extreme, could be defined as the ability of the patient to understand the situation in which he finds himself. It is very important to bear in mind that each subject is, in principle, competent and capable, including the elderly, the mentally ill, adolescents and even preadolescents. In Spain, for example, whenever it is considered that a subject may be unable to make decisions, these decisions will be made by the patient's next of kin or persons close to the patient (article 10 of the Spanish General Health Act) (Simon 1995).

## 2.1 Dimensions of the concept of informed consent

We may identify three basic dimensions of informed consent on the basis of the various definitions: 1) prerequisites such as information, competence, understanding, willingness and voluntariness or lack of coercion; 2) decision-making activities; and 3) outcomes of decision-making (Figure 8).

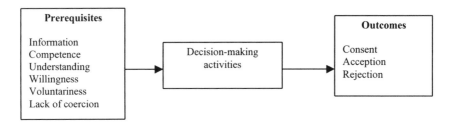

**Figure 8.** Basic dimensions of informed consent

Information is an important precondition for informed consent; people can give informed consent only if they have sufficient information (Davies 1983). It is evident then that the term "informed consent" includes two parties. The first party is a person or persons who offer (Gillett 1989) or disclose information to a patient (Meisel & Roth 1981, Sorrell 1991, Aiken & Catalano 1994, Beauchamp & Childress 1994). It has been observed that the information offered should be sufficient (Aiken & Catalano 1994, Segest 1995), accurate (Gillett 1989) and adequate (Gillon 1986, Gillett 1989, Schachter et al. 1994). Adequate information includes details on the benefits and risks of the proposed and alternative treatments, including the option of no treatment (Schachter et al. 1994). It should also contain details on the nature of the patient's medical condition and the benefits of the proposed treatment or procedure, the risks involved in accepting the proposed treatment or procedure, the significant available alternatives, and the consequences of opting for no treatment or procedure. Further, information should be provided by the person who is responsible for performing the procedure or providing the treatment, generally the physician (Aiken & Catalano 1994).

Faden & Beauchamp (1986) have outlined three criteria for informed consent. The first criterion is that a person must consent on the basis of an understanding of the information. Rowson (1993) observes that it is not enough to provide adequate information, it is also necessary to ensure that the information is understood by the recipient. This draws a distinction between informed consent and educated consent (Rumbold 1996). Educated consent involves a person delivering information in an easily understandable way, as well as ensuring that the patient has understood the information before obtaining consent (see de la Calle et al. 1999). A person who is receiving information should be a competent one, who is able to understand the information received (Meisel & Roth 1981, Sprung & Winic 1989, Beauchamp & Childress 1994, British Medical Association 1995). The second criterion for consent is that consent must not be controlled by influences that might engineer the outcome. This means that it is wrong to withhold any such information from the patient that may discourage the patient from giving consent. The third criterion for consent is that consent must be the intentional giving of permission for an intervention.

A person has to be willing to make a choice (British Medical Association 1995). For the patient to make a reasoned decision he or she must be free to decide one way or the other for his or her own reasons and thus there must be a lack of coercion in the doctor-patient relationship. Although the difference between coercion and persuasion is not clear-cut, it can be said that persuasion aims to enlist the patient's reason by providing information and coercion aims to manipulate the patient's decision by influences which undermine independent reasoning (Gillet 1989).

Freedom is a central prerequisite for informed consent. The crucial question here is voluntariness (Meisel & Roth 1981, Gillon 1986, Dyer & Bloch 1987, Sprung & Wininck 1989), which is associated with a lack of coercion (Gillett 1989). Consent is "a voluntary and continuing permission ... to receive a particular treatment, based on an adequate knowledge of the purpose, nature, likely effects and risks of that treatment, including the likelihood of its success and any alternatives to it" (Department of Health and Welsh Office 1994). For example, Gillon (1986, also Simon 1995) has defined consent as a voluntary, uncoerced decision, made by a sufficiently competent or autonomous person on the basis of adequate information and deliberation, to accept rather that reject some proposed course of action that will affect him or her. According to Simon (1995), consent which is given by a person in order to be subjected to something is only accepted if it is freely given and voluntarily accepted. It is no surprise then that giving consent prior to any health care procedure has been said to be a vital expression of the patient's autonomy (e.g. Draper 1998).

Decision-making activities are a central issue in giving consent (Gillon 1986, Gillett 1989, Sprung & Winick 1989, Aiken & Catalano 1994, Sainz et al. 1994). On the basis of a concept analysis of consent, Brennan (1997) concluded, firstly, that there needs to be a proposed course of action suggested by another party. Secondly, a person needs to have autonomy or be self-governing. Thirdly, a person needs to have a choice from more than one option. Fourthly, a person requires information from which to make that choice. Fifth, a person needs to understand the implications of the decision being made. And lastly, the person must agree to the proposed course of action (Brennan 1997). As an outcome of decision-making, then, a person can accept or reject suggested interventions (Gillon 1986, Aiken & Catalano 1994).

## 3. Realisation of informed consent

### 3.1 Factors supporting informed consent

In order to evaluate the realisation of informed consent in practice, we need to be aware of the factors that affect and that are associated with supporting informed consent in health care. The discussion below will be looking at different types of informed consent and at different ways in which health care personnel can obtain patient's consent (Figure 9). We then move on to discuss the meaning of the quality of the information given and how different norms can support the realisation of informed consent.

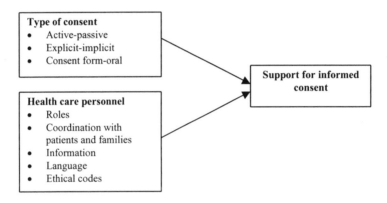

**Figure 9.** Factors supporting informed consent

There are different ways in which informed consent is realised in everyday practice. Informed consent can first of all be defined on the dimensions of activity - passivity. Segest (1995) says that informed consent can be divided into two different phases, information and consent. The first is a more passive act, the second a more active aspect. On the other hand, in medical and nursing care, the purpose of informed consent is to provide clients with a basis for participation in medical decisions (Barnes et al. 1998). This will be done in physician-patient discussions about the risks, benefits and alternatives for treatments (Jablonski et al. 1991). Therefore, informed consent can be seen as a relationship between different parties.

Consent can be explicit or implicit (British Medical Association 1995). Explicit informed consent is usually given by written or verbal agreement, and therefore it is expressed and withdrawn in a formal manner (Bard 1990, UKCC 1992). The signed consent form is the official instrument for obtaining consent. Before the consent form is signed, it is the duty of the doctor to assess the patient for any contraindications, or to see if the patient's condition will add to the risks. If there are any contraindications, this should be told to the medical staff, and any additional risks should be told to the patient (Sidaway v Board of Governors of the Bethlem Royal Hospital and the Maudsley Hospital 1984).

Ideally, the physician will have the patient sign the consent-to-treatment form at the time as the proposed treatment is being discussed. In practice, however, this rarely happens. Typically, the patient is seen in the physician's office where treatments are discussed. The patient will subsequently be admitted to hospital where a nurse will asks him or her to sign a preprinted consent form stating that he or she has been thoroughly informed and has consented to the proposed treatment (Aiken & Catalano 1994). Dimond (1995) suggests that it is better to obtain at least verbal consent from a patient in order for treatment to be carried out, to ensure that all parties are aware of what is being requested. According to Aiken & Catalano (1994), although express consent can be oral or written, written consent is preferable because of the difficulty of proving oral consent.

Implicit consent means that consent is given not just by what we say but also by what we do. Implicit consent is where we go to consult the doctor, describe what is wrong with us, or even roll up our sleeve to allow an examination, e.g. for blood pressure to be measured. Obviously, our consent only covers specific examinations or treatment done at that point and nothing else (Bard 1990). In practice, consent is assumed by, for example, the opening of the mouth for examination, the offering of an arm for taking blood pressure or by attending a doctor and giving information about an illness (British Medical Association 1995). Further, implied consent is non-verbal, e.g. rolling up a sleeve for an injection. However, as this type of consent is non-verbal, there may be a misunderstanding regarding the intended procedure. Therefore it is better to obtain verbal consent from the patient (Dimond 1995).

Consent also has legal connotations. To be legally effective, consent to treatment must be what the law considers "informed consent". This means that the physician or health care practitioner has given the patient enough information regarding the risks and benefits of the proposed treatment and its alternative for the patient to make an intelligent or "informed" decisions (Aiken & Catalano 1994). Further, consent allied to the term informed means that patients should be given the amount of information needed to make an informed choice about a given treatment or intervention (Brennan 1997). Legally, informed consent is a risk management tool that functions essentially as release from liability.

However, there are several problems when obtaining informed consent in practice. One of these arises with the definition of "continuing permission", since the patient can withdraw consent at any point in the treatment process. Another problem is how to define "adequate information". A further problem with the definition of informed consent is that it is unclear what is meant by a "sufficiently competent or autonomous person". This definition compels the health professional to decide who is and who isn't competent to consent to treatment, and thus he/she risks depriving the patient of his/her autonomy. Overall then, it should be perfectly clear that consent is not a clear-cut concept.

Thus, as Simón (1995) states, informed consent is a process. It is not an isolated fact within the relationship between the health worker and user, but a process of meeting and talking between the health worker and the patient which spans the period from when the health worker is in contact with the patient until he is finally released from medical care.

The different roles of persons taking a patient's informed consent have been widely discussed in the literature. There are different views as to whose is the main role in the consent process. According to Segest (1995), the physician's goal in informed consent is not to minimise liability, but to help the patient make the best decision. According to Aiken & Catalano (1994), if consent is not implied or waived, it is the responsibility of the person performing the procedure, usually the physician or surgeon, to obtain the patient's informed consent. Nurse practitioners, however, are responsible for obtaining informed consent when they perform procedures.

The nursing literature, on the other hand, has highlighted the risk of sidelining the concept of consent as a concept affecting doctors only. In terms of what skills the practitioner may need to achieve, assessment skills are important for the nurse to be assured that the person is competent to give consent (Brennan 1997). The realisation of informed consent may be supported by the nurse, and many researchers have described the role of a nurse in the process of informed consent. Davis and Underwood (1989), for example, state that even though nurses are not directly responsible for a client's signature on a medical consent form, in practice they are often asked to obtain this. Nurses can and should be a partner to the patient and the family in the informed consent process by assisting them to be as self-determining as they desire, rather than conforming out of habit, defence or inexperience (e.g. Gadow 1989a,b, Varriccio & Jassak 1989).

Further, nurses need to be aware of patients' rights in the ongoing process of consenting to treatment, not only when signing the form (Barnes et al. 1998). The roles for nurses in informed consent includes the following (Hamaguchi 1998): 1) support of patients' decision-making, 2) promotion of patients' understanding of their own situation, 3) coordination with patients and families, 4) education for health promotion, and 5) taking care of ethical issues.

One of the most important areas where nurses can support the realisation of informed consent in practice is that of information. According to Fry (1989), by understanding the functions and elements of informed consent, nurses can assist their patients to ask for and to comprehend the information they need to be truly and fully informed about treatment choices. She also argues that assessing the risks and benefits of an experimental treatment option may be important to the long-term health of patients. Nurses can also assist patients' decision-making and the assessment of relevant risks and benefits by being fully informed about the planned activities and by applying knowledge of ethical principles to patient care (see also Plank 1994, Simón 1995).

Young (1994) offers four possible actions by which nurses can help the patient as an advocate to avoid litigation. Firstly, the nurse can clarify information already given, as the patient may be in an anxious state when the doctor gives information, and may misinterpret or not hear what has been said. Secondly, the nurse can give the patient extra, non-medical information, and assist the patient to reach a decision. Thirdly, the nurse could give the patient additional medical information, but only if she is sure of the facts and if she is experienced in that area of work. One problem here is that this may not be in accordance with the doctor's wishes; the nurse may be disciplined for going against the doctor's wishes. The risk of discipline must be accepted if the nurse feels strongly that the patient has the right to face certain facts. Finally, as a patient advocate, the nurse is to help the patient formulate and then ask appropriate questions of the doctor. (Young 1994.)

Further, if the doctor has not informed the patient, or refuses to answer the patient's questions, the nurse should take steps, through the chain of command, to ensure that the appropriate person has the physician fulfil his or her responsibility to obtain consent. The physician owes a legal duty to the patient and must act within the acceptable standards to give the information to the patient to meet that legal duty. This duty should not be delegated to the nurse or any other third party (Aiken & Catalano 1994).

The language used in consent forms should be helpful and understandable to the patient, and complex medical and legal terminology should be avoided (Herbert 1980, Simón 1995). During the informed consent process, the patient must also be afforded the opportunity to ask questions. This allows the patient the chance to independently sort out crucial issues before making an informed decision (Plumeri 1994).

Ethical codes (e.g. UKCC 1992) and acts can also support patients' informed consent. Some countries may have specific persons whose role it is to support patients' rights. In Finland, for example, these are ombudsmen who operate on the basis of the Act on the Status and Rights of Patients (785/92).

Spanish nurses have shown little interest in the theory of informed consent, probably because of its recent history (Simón & Barrio 1995). However, nurses have a special ethical responsibility to constantly monitor their patients' information and consent situation (see ethical codes). In Spain, the legal role of the nurse with respect to informed consent is not entirely established and it is disassociated from that of the doctor. However, nurses have much to offer to patients with respect to informed consent: they can collaborate in the evaluation of the degree to which patient consent is voluntary; in the determination of the patient's competence/capacity; in the evaluation of the amount of information that has not been disclosed; in the evaluation of the real understanding that the patient possesses with respect to the information provided, highlighting confusing questions and unclear terms; in the determination of the degree of validity and authenticity of a given consent; and in the development and design of the consent forms (Simón & Barrio 1995).

## 3.2 Factors restricting informed consent

Informed consent in health care is restricted by a variety of different factors. It is generally accepted that a competent adult has the right to consent or to refuse any medical or surgical treatment. However, this "right" is not absolute. For example, courts of law in the US have not allowed patients in certain cases involving minor children, mental illness and substance abuse to refuse life-saving treatments (Aiken & Catalano 1994).

Everyday practice involves a number of restricting factors. These are here divided into four groups: factors associated with a patient him- or herself, factors associated with health care personnel, factors associated with relationships between patient and health care personnel and environmental factors (Figure 10).

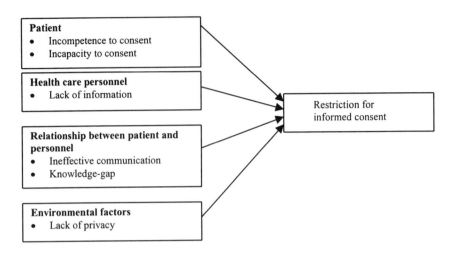

**Figure 10.** Factors restricting informed consent

One of the patient-related factors is competence. From a competence point of view it seems that consent is not a universal human right. The option to give consent can only be given to someone who is deemed to be competent to make decisions affecting their lives. This competence is socially determined and, therefore, by its nature, dynamic and difficult to define (Brennan 1997). The measures of competence that we use today and have used in the past are subjective and change over time (Fulbrook 1994).

Competence to consent is most typically defined as the capacity to comprehend relevant information, the ability to weigh the benefits and risks of the proposed procedure, and the capacity to reach a reasonable decision. While it is important for subjects to remember that they are participating in treatment or research, recall of information is not usually considered to be a valid criterion. Poor recall may be more indicative of the normal forgetting process rather than of incompetence (Stanley et al. 1984). For example, a critically ill patient may be unable to be informed or to consent. The interest of society in promoting health and in acting in the best interest of patients unable to make health decisions for themselves are reflected in the exceptions to the informed consent doctrine (Sprung & Winick 1989). Further, a patient may be anxious, and anxiety is a barrier to communication. Thus, the patient may not be able to take in all that is said to him/her. Indeed, it has been found that in consultations much information is lost, either through a lack of understanding or forgetting on the part of the patient (Ley 1982).

A refusal of consent should be respected, even if it is based on an irrational decision, if it is derived from long-held beliefs and values, on the basis of which a person has run his/her life, but not if the decision is based on a temporary delusion (Kennedy 1992). However, there is a problem here in determining what is an "irrational" decision. There is also the risk that it will be the mentally impaired and demented patients who will be seen to be irrational. When a patient is incompetent to give informed consent, health care decisions can be made by a surrogate decision-maker, someone the patient designated before becoming incompetent (Aiken & Catalano 1994).

Patient refusal may involve various problems. Health professionals in general are not used to having their services refused. When patients refuse to give consent to treatment, staff are usually shocked (Fromer 1981). This, it has been suggested, is because health professionals themselves work in a hierarchic structure in which staff are used to receiving and carrying out instructions from those above them, and giving instructions to those below them. The doctor often feels that he/she knows what is best for the patient, as they have more knowledge than the patient, so a refusal of consent is viewed as a criticism of professional competence.

Dworkin (1988) has highlighted four exceptions where treatment can be given to a patient without obtaining their consent. Firstly, a patient can be treated in an emergency situation without obtaining consent, although, if possible, it is usual to wait until the person has regained consciousness to give consent before treatment is given. Also, treatment without consent can be given when the patient is psychotic, senile, an infant, or otherwise not in a position to give consent. Further, treatment without consent can be given where the patient has specifically asked the doctor not to consult him/her regarding treatment decisions. Finally, treatment without consent can be given when the doctor decides that obtaining informed consent would be harmful to the patient (known as the 'therapeutic privilege' e.g. Canterbury v Spence 1972). However, there is the risk that the plea of therapeutic privilege may conceal an element of unjustified paternalism (Tingle & Cribb 1995).

Restrictive factors may also have to do with the relationship of communication between professional and patient. If this communication is ineffective, the practitioner has failed in his or her role as a responsible counsellor. Health professionals may also use incomprehensible terms and fail to allow the patient clearly to understand his or her condition. Further, there may be a knowledge-gap between doctor and patient. Lastly, if the patient is ill, he or she may be cognitively disadvantaged by more than just a disparity of knowledge. There is broad recognition of the difficulties involved in the sober assessment of one's own illness or those which afflict loved ones. The difficulties induced by illness itself are compounded if there is a lack of trust between doctor and patient as the patient cannot achieve any understanding unless some things at least are believed (Gillett 1989). In addition, the paternalistic tendency assumes either that patients do not want information, or that they would be incapable of understanding it (Byrne et al. 1988, Lavelle-Jones et al. 1993).

It is difficult to make sure that the patient has adequate basic knowledge. The patient may feel that he or she is in a state of dependence on the doctor, which will influence his or her possibility to choose freely (Jensen 1990). In spite of the doctor's best efforts the particular problems of a given patient may not fit into the general summary of facts about the type of condition concerned (Gillet 1989). A further difficulty with informed consent is that even when a patient is told everything appropriate, he or she may not necessarily remember that which he or she, consciously or unconsciously, does not wish to remember (Herbert 1980).

Finally, obtaining consent often happens on hospital wards where other patients may overhear the consultation. This lack of privacy may make patients feel helpless and unable to assert themselves enough to make a decision. It must be realised that although they think the doctor knows what is best for the patient in medical terms (Weiss 1985), it is the nurse who is in regular contact with the patient, and doctors often obtain information about the patient via the nurse. It might be beneficial to involve nurses more closely in medical decisions regarding patients.

## 4. Informed consent in empirical studies

### *4.1 General*

There are number of empirical studies related to informed consent:

> - Consent forms and their understandability
> - Roles of professionals in consent process
> - Emotional factors
> - Cultural issues
> - Information and truth-telling
> - Different clinical areas
> - Patient satisfaction

*Consent forms and their understandability*

Other examples are studies concerned with do-not-resuscitate status (e.g. Russell et al. 1991, Jezewski et al. 1993), paediatric care (e.g Benfield et al. 1991), the security of information management and technology in organisations (e.g. Tonks 1993), end-of-life issues (e.g. Norup et al. 1998), physicians' opinions about ethical issues and informed consent (Sriram et al. 1989) or cultural questions.

Kaufman (1983) has documented the development of the research literature on patient decision-making and informed consent to medical treatment. The analysis covers the literature in three fields of research between 1960 and 1980: medicine, law and the social sciences. Almost 80 % of the articles on consent to medical treatment and research were published in medical journals. The primary concern was with the use of human subjects in medical experimentation and clinical trials. The question of consent to treatment emerged later on. Kaufman also found that most writers contributing to the medical literature were not specialists in medical ethics, nor did they demonstrate sustained work on the topic of patient decision-making; they were researchers or practising physicians from established medical specialities with some interest in examining a topical issue affecting their work.

It has also been stressed in the literature that information including written consent forms should be understandable for persons signing the consent form. According to this basic assumption, readability of informed consent forms has been one central topic in empirical studies (Hammerschmidt & Keane 1992, Zanecchia 1992, Rivera et al. 1992, Grossman et al. 1994, Jubelirer et al. 1994). Many studies have found that much of the written health education materials in the US is not understandable to patients (e.g. Grundner 1980, Morrow 1980, Streiff 1986, Dixon & Park 1990, Michielutte et al. 1990).

The readability of informed consent forms describing clinical oncology protocols at one oncology centre in the US were assessed in the study by Grossman et al. (1994). Three readability indices (the Flesch Reading Ease Score, the Flesch-Kincaid Formula, the Robert Gunning Fog Index) were used in the study which comprised 137 consent forms. The results suggested that the consent forms were written at a level that is difficult for most patients to read, despite national, cooperative group, institutional and departmental review. The authors suggest that the consent process should be strengthened by improving the readability of the forms. Similar results were reported in a study by Hammerschmidt and Keane (1992), who analysed 65 consent forms. Most of them were complex enough to be comprehensible to only a minority of patients (also Jubelirer et al. 1994). The readability of consent forms used in contraceptive clinical trials has also been found to be poor. The most common problems seem to be the use of unfamiliar or long words and long sentences (Rivera et al. 1992).

However, not all countries have conducted readability studies on consent forms. In Spain, for example, Simon et al. (1996) state simply that the written informed consent forms used can be comprehended, but until recently no adequate instruments have been available for measuring this. It is indeed essential to make the written forms used easier to understand if the aim is to guarantee the ethical quality of the process of informed consent.

*Roles of professionals in consent process*

Empirical research has also been done into the roles of different persons. Mark & Spiro (1990) evaluated and compared the informed consent of 102 out-patients and their physicians (n = 16) to undergo a colonoscopy. The physicians said more often that the decision to have the colonoscopy had been made by the patient or had been shared, while patients disagreed and held the physician most responsible for the decision. Silva (1985) assessed the adequacy of 75 spouses' comprehension of the information needed to give informed consent to participate in research. She found that spouses had adequate comprehension of the information needed.

*Emotional factors*

Informed consent causes emotionally difficult situations for personnel. For example, Stolman et al. (1994) studied physicians' and residents' (n = 158) attitudes and factors affecting autopsy consent. Physicians generally find it difficult to deal with the emotional issues of death and dying and entering into discussions concerned with obtaining autopsy permission. 39 % of 80 respondents said that they always or sometimes find it difficult to notify the family when a child whom they are caring for dies, while 41 % said they always find it stressful to ask permission for autopsy. Fourteen of 76 indicated that they do not ask permission for autopsy if the family is angry or upset. When asking why physicians request permission for autopsy in a half-hearted manner, 36

% of 104 respondents ranked as most important the physician's belief that the family would be upset at the request. The second most important factor mentioned by 19 respondents was the belief that little or no important information would be obtained. In a open-ended question, 46 of 75 respondents indicated that the best time to ask permission for autopsy is immediately or several hours after the death of the patient, while 12 believed that the best time is before the patient dies.

Ethical dilemmas relating to informed consent were also uncovered in Davis's (1989) study. Responses to vignettes and semi-structured interviews with nurses ( n = 27) pointed to dilemmas of structural philosophical influences relating to informed consent. Structural influences included considerations such as type and location of institution, organisation of work, institutional policies and procedures, and accountability structure. Philosophical influences refer to implicit epistemologic positions held by nurses.

*Cultural issues*

Informed consent is an important tool with which health care personnel can assure patients' participation in treatment in different cultures (see Cross & Churchill 1982). Tajima (1997) mentioned that the idea of informed consent and promotion of better communication between patients and physician seems to be particularly important for Japanese physicians. In India, Sriram et al. (1989) conducted a study into physicians' opinions on ethical issues in medical research. The majority of the respondents (n = 629) noted the relevance of ethics in different medical situations, though in certain areas (such as community health and research using animals) ethical issues were felt to be less important. Nearly half of the respondents have obtained oral consent only and physicians have noted a strong need for an orientation course in medical ethics. Newton et al. (1994) examined Indian academic and private practice physicians' (n = 81) opinions about informed consent. Opinions varied among physicians as to whether patients must be informed of the potential need for surgery, prolonged hospital stay, or death relating to endoscopic retrograde cholangiopancreatography. The performing physicians felt they were ultimately responsible for obtaining consent. Only 4 - 22 % of the respondents felt that a registered nurse, alone or with the assistance of a secretary, intern, resident or primary-care physician, was adequate in the informed consent process. Less that 11 % felt that the registered nurse alone should obtain consent.

Not all medical doctors are aware of the informed consent document, however. This was discovered in study conducted in Spain; 59.4 % of 130 medical doctors were aware of the informed consent document, 39 % knew only little about its content. 30.9 % thought that the document could help to improve the relationship between doctor and patient, 16 % thought this relationship could even deteriorate (Viñas et al. 1999).

Cultural differences have also been highlighted in studies which document variation in expectations and in the implementation of informed consent, advance directives and life-sustaining treatment practices across different cultures (Kaufert & O'Neil 1990, Muller & Desmond 1992). In the study by Barnes et al. (1998), the sample consisted of Latino, Chinese and Anglo-American cancer patients in the US. Data collection included open-ended, in-depth interviews, observations and reviews of charts and other clinical documents. There were problems in language and communication and the health care providers were not sure about the level of understanding of their clients. The busy climate of the hospital and clinic, coupled with multiple health care providers working with clients, limits and constrains the type and amount of information that is communicated, including the information that a patient requires to be fully informed and to make decisions. Some patients seemed to be passive about medical decisions because of a lack of choices. Others were passive, choosing to relegate decision-making to the professionals. There were differences in how much the patients wanted to be involved in decisions. Therefore, the degrees of desired control over decision-making may vary according to the patient's gender, culture, age, past experiences or expertise at making decisions, as well as to the duration and intensity of the patient-provider relationship (Wiens 1993, Barnes et al. 1998).

*Information and truth-telling*

Informed consent has to do with information and truth-telling. Pang (1998) analysed the moral tension of nurses in China concerning the practice of informed consent. Nurses in China have a moral obligation to treat patients with sincerity, which carries a strong sense of parental protectiveness. Therefore, nurses in China are ambivalent about the notion of truthfulness. It was found that most nurses would prefer to tell the truth to patients, but their primary ethical justification is not the respect of patients' autonomy or safeguarding patients' right of self-determination. Nurses' interventions are rather beneficent in nature, and they base their decisions to reveal the truth on whether or not patients will receive more relevant treatment and better nursing care.

Dalla-Vorgia et al. (1992) studied the attitudes of Greeks to truth-telling. 500 questionnaires were gathered from apparently healthy people who either visited a health centre, were members of a friendship club in Athens, attended a seminar in health statistics or in epidemiology or public health. The respondents were asked three main questions: 1) if someone is seriously ill and it is certain that he or she will soon die, should the doctor tell the truth; 2) if someone is seriously ill and it is very probable that he or she will die, but not very soon, should the doctor tell the truth; not; and 3) if someone is seriously ill and has a relatively low probability of dying, should the doctor tell the truth. The preset options were: yes, no, and it depends. As far as the Greeks are concerned, the decision on whether or not to tell the truth "depends": it depends on age, education, family status, occupation, place of birth and residence and on whether or not they are religious people. However, it does not depend on their sex. The authors conclude that doctors should not lie, but should disclose to their patients that part of the truth they are ready to accept.

*Different clinical areas*

Sorrell (1991) addressed the question of whether writing or speaking about information in an informed consent document helps patients in an X-ray department of an urban hospital comprehend information related to their informed participation in a health education programme. A post-test only control-group design was used with 80 volunteers. They were randomly assigned to three groups: writing group, speaking group or comparison group. Participants were read the informed consent document while waiting for a scheduled mammogram. Those in the writing group wrote their responses to the questions: what do you remember about what you read; what two additional things do you want to know more about; and what concerns do you have about participating in this project. In the speaking group, subjects were allowed 15 minutes to respond orally to the same three questions. The comparison group were not asked to write or speak about the information given in the informed consent document. All subjects completed post-test questionnaires approximately 45 minutes after reading the informed consent document. Comparison of the results for the three groups indicated that writing and speaking may be efficient and effective interventions in the informed consent process.

There are also studies which suggest that the level of stress and anxiety may increase with more information (e.g. Lalli 1980, Lalli & Greenstreet 1981). Hopper et al. (1994) studies a total of 1251 patients who were given IV injections. Among the patients awaiting the administration of IV contrast material, those awaiting the administration of ionic contrast material who were not informed of the risks showed a statistically significantly higher risk of an elevated anxiety score.

Edwards et al. (1998) reviewed 812 articles to study different methods of obtaining informed consent. Out of these articles 14 provided comparative data on different methods of obtaining informed consent. These studies were then classified according to three outcome measures: anxiety, consent rate and understanding. The results suggest that giving people more information and more time to reflect tends to be associated with a lower consent rate. More information seems to be associated with greater awareness of the research nature of the trial, voluntary participation, right to withdraw and available alternative treatments. There was evidence of an interaction with knowledge: high levels of knowledge are significantly associated with less anxiety, irrespective of consent method.

Patients' awareness of the risks of radiological examination has also been studied. Patients (n = 160) were randomised into two groups and they were provided with either written or computer-based (video) informed consent. Female patients in the video group scored better results in the test than those in the group with the written consent form. By contrast, no differences were found between men in the two groups. In practice it took the patients longer to complete the video informed consent form (Hopper et al. 1994).

Informed consent questions have been related to different interventions such as patient transfers (e.g. Kellermann & Ackerman 1988, Jablonski et al. 1991). Kellermann and Ackerman (1988) offer four reasons why transfer patients are entitled to informed consent: 1) patients have a right to emergency treatment that can be waived only with the patient's informed consent, 2) the patient's well-being is protected by informed consent, 3) physician and institutional accountability for transfer decisions is raised by requiring informed consent and 4) patients are assured of being adequately informed of their rights. Further, the purpose of the study by Jablonski et al. (1991) was to evaluate whether informed consent was obtained prior to transfers of patients from a community hospital to a Veterans' affairs medical centre in the US. There were 86 consecutive interhospital-transferred patients in the study, and also physicians were interviewed. Informed consent was reported for none of the transfers by patient interview, compared with 11 % of the transfers assessed by physician interviews. The risks of transfer were discussed infrequently according to both physicians (17 %) and patients (13 %). Physicians recalled discussing the benefits of the transfer more frequently than did patients (80 % vs. 42 %). Physicians also recalled discussing alternatives to transfer more frequently than did patients (61 % vs. 18 %). The authors conclude that verbal informed consent is obtained infrequently prior to interhospital transfer and that the risks of transfers are seldom perceived and discussed with patients.

In radiology, professionals increasingly obtain information consent for the IV injection of contrast medium, with more than half currently requesting consent from their patients (Lambe et al. 1992). Most patients want to be informed of the risks associated with ionic contrast material before its administration (Winfield et al. 1986, Spring et al. 1988, Hopper et al. 1992). Further, the average patient is not knowledgeable about all risks associated with the use of IV contrast material. Patients with more than a high-school level of education and who had previously received contrast material scored better results with regard to understanding the risks associated with the use of contrast material (Neptune et al. 1994).

Elements of informed consent in clinical research with drugs were surveyed with 302 Spanish clinical investigators in order to determine whether the patient's information sheet should be prepared for each trial and what items of information should be included. Ninety-one percent the investigators considered it necessary to prepare a patient's information sheet for each clinical trial. At least 83 % considered that the following information should always be included: an invitation to participate in a clinical trial, the aims of the study, a description of the predictable benefits and risks, a declaration that participation is voluntary and a statement that refusal does not affect normal medical care. Only 29 % and 53 % thought that patients should always be informed about the clinical trial design and data confidentiality. (Dal-Ré 1992.)

*Patient satisfaction*

One closely related research area is that concerned with patient satisfaction. Many satisfaction studies point at problems with patient information, which seems to be the most common reason for dissatisfaction (e.g. MacDaniel & Nash 1990, Leino-Kilpi & Vuorenheimo 1992, Bond & Thomas 1992, Thomas & Bond 1996, O'Malley 1997). Recent satisfaction studies have included comparisons of patient satisfaction with treatment in different European countries (WHO 1996a). A study by the WHO indicated that overall, satisfaction with health care in Eastern Europe is relatively high, although a North-South divide is evident. Greeks, Italians, Spanish and Portuguese people show high levels of dissatisfaction. This concerns not only the quality of care, but also issues of efficiency and organisation. The picture is exactly the opposite in northern countries, where 90 % indicate high levels of satisfaction (WHO 1996a).

## 4.2 Informed consent and care of the elderly and chronically ill

Sugarman et al. (1998) provide an excellent overview of empirical research into informed consent and care of the elderly and chronically ill. The primary goal of their review was to gain a deeper understanding of the particular challenges involved in obtaining meaningful informed consent from older adults. The literature review was based on 10 databases. The total of 99 articles and 289 unique research questions covered a wide range of aspects of informed consent: recruitment (60), decision-making capacity (21), voluntariness (6), disclosure (30), understanding (139), consent forms (7) authorisation (11), policies (13) and other (2). In this review recruitment was analysed in relationship to informed consent. The results were mixed: some studies demonstrated that older age was associated with a lower participation rate in research, or had no association with the participation rate. No evidence was found that older age correlated with increased participation (Sugarman et al. 1998).

Decision-making capacity has been evaluated either on a more general level or against a more particular capacity criterion. The particular criteria evaluated for assessing decision-making capacity included the rationality of choice, patient's appreciation of illness, understanding, evidence of a choice and reasonableness of choice. However, none of these simple criteria performed well as a screening test or surrogate for a formal evaluation of decision-making capacity (Sugarman et al. 1998).

In voluntariness, Sugarman et al. (1998) identified just a few research questions. In disclosure studies, there are two areas: attitudes towards disclosure and the content of disclosure itself. Many patients are satisfied with the information given, but others want more. Also, it seems that healthy persons get more information than cancer patients, older patients are told less than younger ones. Multiple methods enhance the completeness of disclosure and resident physicians typically disclose more information than nurses or the attending physician staff. Understanding was the most common area in the analysis. A substantial number of studies with different populations showed that increased age was related to diminished comprehension. These populations included those with serious mental illnesses, community dwellers, cardiac catheterisation patients, colonoscopy patients, surgery patients, voluntarily admitted psychiatric patients, nursing home patients given clinical vignettes and cardiac patients in a clinical trial. Studies in informed consent forms demonstrate that simpler presentations in forms improve comprehension. There are also other studies which have demonstrated that typical consent forms are very difficult to understand, especially for the elderly (Sugarman et al. 1998).

Drawing on their extensive literature review, Sugarman et al. (1998) conclude that some aspects of the informed consent process have received considerable attention in studies with older adults, others have not. Older age and less formal education are clearly associated with impaired understanding of informed consent information. Therefore, it is very important to determine whether elderly patients can make competent decisions (e.g. understand treatment information) concerning medical care. If some of these patients are found to be incapable, acceptable procedures for substitute decision-making should be considered (Stanley et al. 1984).

Little has been written specifically about the medical and nursing care of elderly people with dementia from the perspective of consent to treatment (Watson 1994).

Indeed, the competency of the aged, as a group, has been the subject of some controversy, and opinions vary widely as to the capabilities of the older population. On the other hand, elderly patients are often viewed as a highly heterogeneous group who cannot be classifies as a distinct group (Stanley et al. 1984).

Stanley et al. (1984) evaluated geriatric patients' capacity to consent to research. Competence was investigated through the use of hypothetical consent information on three dimensions: comprehension of consent material, quality of reasoning about the decision to participate or not participate in research, and reasonable choice regarding participation. They found that elderly patients' choices about those projects in which participation is 'reasonable' did not differ from younger patients. However, the elderly showed significantly poorer comprehension of consent information.

Fitten and Waite (1990) compared the decision-making capacity of over 60-year-old, presumably competent, hospitalised patients (n = 25) and healthy, age and education matched controls (n = 25). The vignette results indicated a significant difference between study and control groups in understanding key treatment issues: healthy controls demonstrated a better understanding of these issues. The results suggested that presumably competent, medically ill elders may be at risk for developing decisional impairments during hospitalisation. The researchers concluded that obtaining informed consent directly from many of these patients may not be feasible.

It has been suggested that a simplified, illustrated storybook format is useful in conveying relevant information to the elderly (e.g. Tymchuk et al. 1986, Tymchuk & Ouslander 1990, Ouslander et al. 1993, Krynski et al. 1994). This type of information was used in a study of elderly people's decision-making about tube feeding. It showed that there are no differential increases in anxiety as a result of explicit discussion about the consequences of tube feeding (Krynski et al. 1994). However, it is not clear whether when an individual chooses to have or reject a life-sustaining intervention in an advance directive, the person does so by making a truly informed decision (Kayser-Jones 1990).

Blackhall et al. (1995) studies truth-telling to very old subjects. The oldest subjects (aged 81 years and over) were less likely to believe that the patient should be told the truth about a terminal prognosis than were the youngest subjects. Subjects with personal experience of illness and withholding and withdrawing care were more likely to favour truth-telling. No relationships were found for sex, functional status, or access to care.

## 4.3 Informed consent and acute care

Informed consent has been studied quite often in the context of acute care, especially in connection with operative activities and anaesthesia (e.g. Clark et al. 1991, Lonsdale & Hutchison 1991, Inglis & Farnill 1993, Vessey & Siriwardena 1998). Herz et al. (1992) say that related questions began to attract considerable interest in neurosurgery in the early 1970s. The complex environment and technology may impair the ability of patients to participate in medical decision-making or to give informed consent (Cohen et al. 1993). Much interest has also been shown in the effects of preoperative information. Some studies support the provision of risk information: it satisfies the legal requirements of informed consent and allows patients the autonomy to make informed choices (Riley & Simmonds 1992).

A number of studies have shown that most patients cope better with stressful medical procedures if they are warned about the distressing aspects of the procedure in advance (e.g. Suls & Wan 1989). However, some patients tend to be "information avoiders" and they may cope better with reduced amounts of information (Shaw et al. 1986).

Dawes et al. (1992) assessed the attitudes of patients (n = 150) towards informed consent using different types of consent interviews. The patients were over 16 years of age, admitted the day before their nose and throat operation (tonsillectomy, intranasal polypectomy, submucosal resection of the nasal septum, septoplasty, intranasal antrostomy) that was to be performed under general anaesthesia. There were three study groups. In Group A, patients had an informal interview prior to giving their consent. In Group B, an information sheet was used to guide the interview with patients before they signed the hospital consent form, and in Group C, the information sheet was read with the patient before they signed the hospital consent form. It was found that most patients were happy to do as their doctor advised. However, they thought that the informal consent interview is important because it gives them information. Patients also wanted to know about most, but not all, complications involved in the procedure. One-quarter worried about the anaesthesia, one-eighth worried about complications and other things such as pain and nausea. Patients who had an informal interview felt obligated to sign the consent form. They also thought it had medico-legal implications. In contrast, those who had a structured interview felt less obligated to sign the consent form and were more involved in the decision to operate.

Some studies point at the difficulties patients have to understand informed consent forms and/or the information give in them (e.g. Muss et al. 1979, Cunningham 1989). However, a study on information provided for cancer patients entering a clinical trial does not lend support to this assumption. Jensen et al. (1993) also found that information given before treatment was well remembered after three months, and detailed information allowed patients to understand and participate in treatment decisions. Further, Cassileth et al. (1980) studied 200 cancer patients being treated by chemotherapy, radiation or surgery. Only 59 % of the patients correctly understood the purpose of their treatment and only 55 % could list one major complication.

Taplin (1995) carried out a study in which a mixed sample of patients were interviewed post-operatively to establish their views on the consent procedure and to find out how much information each had been given, as a basis for making an informed decision about treatment. She conducted interviews with each patient, asking them eight simple questions regarding their treatment and consent. It was found that there was little adequate informed consent, so that the signature itself meant very little. Some of the patients were even unaware of the purpose of the consent form, and many of them were unaware of the operation they had just signed for. This suggests that the explanations offered have been inadequate. It was also found that in many cases, the consent form included incorrect or irrelevant information, or important information had been omitted. It is suggested that the above discrepancies may be due to staff and patients not taking consent seriously enough.

In a study among patients (n = 49) with acute abdominal pain (Vessey & Siriwardena 1998) 42 patients understood why an operation was being planned, but 28 patients stated that there had been no preoperative discussion of any potential side-effects or complications of surgery. The authors suggest that there is a clear need for improved discussion in these areas.

Understanding of the different elements of informed consent was also analysed by 38 consecutive patients admitted to hospital for total joint replacement. Understanding evaluated at the time when they signed the consent document before the operation, their recall of those elements was reviewed six months after the operation. Six months after the operation, the understanding of risks and benefits that had been demonstrated before the operation by both verbal questioning and the signed consent document was compared. At six months, the number of patients who recalled the risks ranged from 25 % who remembered the risk of infection to only one who remembered the risk of damage to a nerve or artery. The numbers who remembers the potential benefits were higher: 22 % for relief of pain and improved function and 16 % for improved motion. Patients who assessed themselves as nervous before the operation tended to remember more during the questioning at the instruction of informed consent. However, their recall six months later was not significantly better (Hutson et al. 1991).

In the study by Clark et al. (1991, see also Leighton et al. 1987) the purpose was to evaluate the effect of a preprinted, risk-specific consent form on the amount of anaesthetic risk information patients retain from the preoperative interview. In the study group there were 92, and in the control group 125 inpatients. Both groups took part in a standard oral discussion covering anaesthetic risk information. In the control group this information was received only orally and patients were interviewed two weeks prior to implementation of a preprinted anaesthesia consent form. Patients in the study group received this information orally and via a preprinted consent form and were interviewed between the fourth and sixth weeks after implementation of a preprinted anaesthesia consent form. The authors found that patients remembered less of the information conveyed during the preoperative interview if they were given the preprinted consent form at the beginning of the interview. Based on the results it was theorised that patients who see an anaesthesia consent form for the first time during the preoperative interview may try to read and listen simultaneously and with their attention divided, may remember less of the preoperative discussion. These authors previously (Leighton et al. 1987) found that surgical outpatients were both more anxious and remembered less of the information presented if they received a preprinted, risk-specific form at the beginning of the preoperative interview, as compared with patients who did not receive such a form. The authors conclude that there is a need to improve the methods of information.

In neurosurgery, Herz et al. (1992) conducted an interesting trial in patient information and teaching. A total of 106 neurosurgical patients were involved in a teaching programme carried out in collaboration between physicians and nurses. According to the results, patients showed the greatest interest in and understanding of diagnoses and surgical techniques. Individuals paid much less attention to risks, which is one of the most crucial topics related to informed consent. Relatively little interest was also demonstrated in post-operative self-care and follow-up in the spirit of collaborative participation with respect to the health care process. In addition, patients' concepts of the goals and benefits of a proposed treatment were relatively poorly understood. In their conclusions the authors highlight various problems in the process of informed consent, such as lack of time to inform patients, the ability of patients to absorb or retain information and the selective memory of patients. These all make the process of informed consent difficult and the outcomes are not clear.

As for factors improving the quality of informed consent, Lavelle-Jones et al. (1993) studied 265 patients undergoing intrathoracic, intraperitoneal and vascular surgical procedures. Of these patients 192 were followed up for six months. The results showed that patients were best informed immediately after signing the consent form; from then on recall of information deteriorated. However, about two-thirds (69 %) of the patients admitted they had not read the consent form before signing it. Elderly patients and those with below-average points in reading tests, impaired cognitive functions, and external locus of control had poor information recall.

A recent study assessing patient anxiety after being informed is that by Kerrigan et al. (1993), who tested the assumption that patients would become unduly anxious if given detailed information about the risks of surgery in an attempt to obtain fully informed consent. Patient anxiety was measured before and after information was given concerning the risks involved. One group of men were given detailed information, another group of men were given a simple explanation of what the surgery involved. A detailed account of the facts did not increase anxiety, and actually had the advantage of allowing patients a fully informed choice before they consented to surgery. Inglis and Farnill (1993), however, suggest that in the Kerrigan et al. (1993) study the design included no checks on whether the information was actually understood by their patients.

Patients' anxiety was also measured in the study by Inglis and Farnill (1993). The patients were randomly allocated to either a routine (n = 20) or a detailed information (n = 20) group. It was found that the provision of detailed information about the risks of general anaesthesia did increase patients' knowledge but did not increase their anxiety. Pain did not interfere with the patients' ability to give informed consent in a study among patients with acute abdominal pain (Vessey & Siriwardena 1998).

Different methods have been used to evaluate whether there is any link between methods used and patients' anxiety level. Four different groups were used in the study by Dawes et al. (1992) to assess patients' anxiety level and recall of the operation name, details of the operation and its complications. Patients in Group A did not have a consent interview until the study was completed; Group B patients had an informal interview prior to giving their consent; patients in Group C got a written sheet to guide the interview with the patients before they signed the hospital consent form; and in Group D the written information sheet was read with the patient before they signed the hospital consent form. It was found that patients had higher than normal anxiety levels when admitted, but several hours later the interview anxiety was normal for Groups B, C, and D; Group A maintained a higher level of anxiety. Only 37 % correctly recalled the operation name, whereas 87 % of all groups recalled the explanation of the operation. However, Groups C and D recalled a higher mean number of complications per patient. The authors conclude that a structured interview, when obtaining informed consent, increases the number of complications recalled without increasing pre-operative anxiety.

Patients' desire for information was analysed in a study by Lonsdale & Hutchison (1991). Patients in Canada (n = 138) and Scotland (n = 49) were asked to complete a pre-operative questionnaire examining their desire for information relating to anaesthesia. In general, Canadians were more positive ("Like to know" or "Right to know") in their desire for information, but the response was very similar. In Canada, more than 90 % of the patients wanted to meet the anaesthetist pre-operatively, wanted to know when they allowed to eat and drink, how long they were anaesthetised, premedicant drugs and when they allowed up. In Scotland, more than 70 % of the patients wanted to meet the anaesthetist pre-operatively, wanted pain relief, wanted to know when allowed to eat and drink and when allowed up. In both countries, patients under the age of 50 years were more positive in their desire for information; neither Canadian or Scottish patients give a high priority to being informed about dangerous complications. The high priority placed on information about time to eating and drinking and mobility suggests that patients are most concerned about a clear timetable to recovery. The authors conclude that detailed information about every aspect of medical care may cause distress to some patients and that further investigation is required to discover whether such information benefits or adversely affects the patients who receive it.

Cohen et al. (1993) compared patients' and nurses' agreement of the intuitive assessment of ICU patients' cognition, judgement and decision-making capacity. In addition they examined whether those assessments agreed with abbreviated formal mental status testing. It was found that residents' and nurses' assessments of cognition and judgement showed a high degree of agreement. In addition, their assessments correlated highly with abbreviated formal mental status testing.

Cobo et al. (1999) studied the attitudes of 133 ICU patients and families towards the informed consent document. They found that 100 % read the document, 95.4 % were satisfied with the verbal information they had received, and 4.6 % were not satisfied. Over four-fifths or 88.8 % of the patients thought that the aim of the document was to inform and to ask for the patient's consent, 12.9 % thought its main aim was to inform and to relieve the doctor's responsibility. De la Calle et al. (1999) studied 935 surgical patients' perceptions of information obtained. 93.3 % said that patients were informed by the medical doctor. Only 4.3 % expressed said that the information was provided by a nurse, 1.2 % by next of kin and 1.1 % by others.

In Sweden, Athlin et al. (1992) conducted a study on information about post-operative information of cancer patients. A total of 64 patients were involved in the study, 32 cancer patients and 36 hernia patients. Cancer patients were given more attention by the medical doctors post-operatively and were given more opportunities to ask about the operation than the hernia patients. However, there was lack of privacy in the information situation and both groups were informed on the ward in the presence of other patients. Houghton et al. (1997) also identified problems in the process of informed consent in the surgery. They say that the important task of obtaining informed consent is often left to the most junior member of the surgical team, whose understanding of surgical procedures involved may be limited.

In Finland, Kanerva et al. (1999) investigated the process of informed consent among day-surgery patients. The research material was collected from four district hospital patients in surgical wards (n = 107). According to the results, 63 % expressed their consent by going to surgery. Oral consent was given by 56 % and written consent by 13 % of the patients. Most had given voluntary consent knowing that they had the opportunity to refuse surgery. Most had also obtained sufficient information about health as well as about the significance and benefits of the operation; one-quarter had not received sufficient information about the risks involved in the surgery and the benefits of the anaesthesia used. However, the patients had not clearly understood the information about the benefits or disadvantages of the anaesthesia in use and any alternative treatments.

*4.4 Informed consent and gynaecological or maternity care*

There is only limited research into questions of informed consent in the context of maternity care. Ethical issues in gynaecological examinations, however, are discussed in the literature related to obstetric ultrasonography (Chernevak & McCullough 1992). The opportunity of women to disagree with their physicians on the need for Caesarean section has also been discussed (Catlin 1998). The lack of empirical research is quite surprising in view of the fact that gynaecological interventions such as abortions are among the most common operations in the world. Some research has been done into women's right to abortion, the rights of the fetus and the rights and duties of physicians and midwives (e.g. Hord & Delano 1994).

In the United Kingdom in 1996, the General Medical Council Standards Committee issued guidelines on intimate examinations (Royal College of Obstetricians and Gynaecologists 1997, Randall 1998). This document was aimed at obstetricians and gynaecologists working in hospital settings, but it is also useful for those working in community settings. These guidelines emphasise the importance of patient information. Professionals should explain to the patient why an intimate examination needs to be done; they should also explain what the examination will involve and obtain the patient's permission. Randall (1998) has described some areas causing concern in these guidelines and provided faculty recommendations. These include that patients should be asked to give verbal consent.

Some studies have also highlighted the importance of discussions on informed consent in gynaecological examinations, e.g. prior to amniocentesis in the ultrasound evaluation (Katz et al. 1991). However, this is not always the case in gynaecological treatment. Sommerseth (1993) surveyed women's (n = 891) perceptions of information provided about routine ultrasound examinations around the 17th week of pregnancy. About half (n = 888, 51 %) said that they had not received any form of information before the ultrasound examination. The authors argue that if a pregnant woman is supposed to make the decision about whether or not to have a prenatal ultrasound scan, she must have specific information to enable her to do so.

In Denmark, legislation obligates the patient and the general practitioner to confirm by their signatures that the patient has received information about sterilisation, its risks and consequences. Rasmussen et al. (1992) asked 97 men and 96 women if they received this information prior to their sterilisation and their knowledge about sterilisation. It was found that 54 % of women and 35 % men indicated they had not received this information. On the other hand, only a few of these patients wanted further information from the hospital doctor, and their knowledge about sterilisation was good. The authors recommend that both the general practitioner and the hospital responsible for the operation ensure that the patient receives optimal information.

In Sweden, a study has been performed to determine whether participants in a gynaecological trial had perceived adequate information according to the guidelines of the Declaration of Helsinki. In this study 43 women out of 53 who completed the trial returned the questionnaire. All but one of the participants had been aware that they were taking part in a research project. However, five said that they had not been aware that a second laparoscopy had been performed for research reasons only; seven had not been aware of the meaning of participating in the project; and 17 said they had no information on being able to withdraw from the study. The authors emphasise the meaning of information quality in informed consent (Lynöe et al. 1991).

Rivera et al. (1992) applied three different methods to evaluate the readability of an informed consent form used in contraceptive clinical trials. The most common problems associated with high readability scores were the use of unfamiliar words, long words and long sentences.

Maternal attitudes in prepared and unprepared Caesarean deliveries were analysed in 143 women. Preparation involved the provision of much information. The results showed that prepared Caesarean women had a significantly greater desire for active participation in the delivery than women unprepared for Caesarean delivery. It seems that preparation and information support an active role and participation (Hart 1980).

Swan and Borshoff (1994) investigated informed consent among 40 primiparous labouring women. Their basic assumption that it is the patient's right to determine whether she will or will not have an epidural inserted for pain relief during labour. Therefore, it is the responsibility of the anaesthetist to provide information to patients so that they can make an intelligent decision. Forty labouring women were given information about the risks of post-epidural puncture headache, post-epidural backache and more serious complications. The women were then surveyed 36 to 48 hours postpartum to assess their recall of the information given. The results showed that the subjects did not recall all the information given afterwards: 67 % of the subjects recalled that epidural risks were discussed, while 33 % could not recall any discussion at all concerning epidural risks; antenatal epidural information classes seem to support recall. The authors conclude that informed consent should be obtained antenatally whenever possible. They also suggest that the informed consent is obtained with both the labouring mother and next-of-kin present.

It is believed that informed consent for epidural analgesia during labour is inadequate and that patients are poorly informed and unable to cope with the information during labour for informed consent. Pattee et al. (1997) surveyed 60 mothers during the first months after vaginal delivery. The mothers considered it important that all information on epidural related complications be disclosed. The level of satisfaction with the consent process was relatively high (8.1/10). Patient satisfaction with the consent process was not affected by opioid premedication, anxiety, pain score, education group or level of pain relief.

# Discussion and conclusion

In this publication, an overview about the concepts of autonomy, privacy and informed consent has been made, based on the existing laws, ethical codes and literature. The purpose is to give a general picture about these concepts, and how they have been empirically investigated in health care. The overview has been made in collaboration between the researchers from five European countries, these are Finland, Germany, Greece, Spain, and the United Kingdom. These countries are part of the BIOMED2-project "Patients' autonomy and privacy in nursing interventions", funded by the European Commission and this report is the first publication of the project.

The overview is based on the existing literature. The main international sources used are Medline and Cinahl-databases, but also legal texts, ethical codes, books and reports have been included. National data differs according to the country and it includes research reports, textbooks and articles. Getting hold of the literature, however, was quite problematic. In each of the concept areas (autonomy, privacy, informed consent) there is a large amount of literature in the main databases. But also in more theoretical articles as well as empirical ones, the focus and structure are not always clear and it is difficult to determine the connection with these concepts. Further, in empirical studies the research questions and data collected are not always clearly described. Thus, a clearly systematic approach was difficult to offer. We hope, however, that the report gives a satisfactory overview in the area and that the list of references itself is useful for readers.

The empirical studies analysed try to refer mainly to the three clinical areas: elderly care, surgical and maternity care. The reason for seeking more information in elderly care, surgical and maternity care was that ongoing research projects concentrates in these areas. Among these, most empirical research has been done in elderly and surgical care, and less in maternity care and in the gynaecological area. However, other areas were also strongly represented in the literature such as internal medicine, critical care units etc. In order to get a more comprehensive view, more clinical specialities should be included in future projects. There is a special need to analyse the most vulnerable groups of patients, e.g. in mental health, paediatrics and care of the disabled (see Brazier & Lobjoit 1991).

Laws and codes represent the strongest part of normative ethics. In many of the countries, the autonomy of patients and/or clients in health care has been included in the laws, either generally or referring to special groups of patients. It is, however, difficult to form a comprehensive picture, because legislative elements in the different countries vary in structure and approach. From five different countries, i.e. Finland, Germany, Greece, Spain, and the United Kingdom, only in Spain and Finland patients' status and rights have been clearly established in a parliamentary act. One conclusion of the present report is: more coherent legislation on patients' rights at the European level is needed. This would ensure equality between patients in different European countries and help professionals when moving from one country to another. As a more practical conclusion, a data base of acts, laws, and professional codes should be established.

Many professional codes in health care are in existence. This can be seen as a symbol of professional status. These codes are similar in content. For example, those for nurses have been influenced by the ethical codes of the International Council of Nurses (1973). In the light of inter-disciplinarity, it should be considered whether the codes of different professionals could be combined into a more comprehensive one. Advantages and disadvantages of such a more general code for different professionals need to be subject of future research.

The concept of autonomy is one of the basic concepts in health care and nursing ethics. A vast body of literature exists about this concept. The literature, however, does not give any precise definition of the concept. Autonomy seems to consist of different dimensions such as perspectives, preconditions, decisions and actions. The existing empirical studies mainly emphasise the dimensions of preconditions and decision-making. The realisation of the concept of autonomy takes place through different human activities. These activities can be either supported or restricted in health care. Supporting factors can be divided into internal (ability and capacity) and external ones. Main restricting internal factors are physical and mental conditions and current preferences; external factors can be social, financial, organisational and informational in nature. Thus, we can conclude that in future, the concept needs a more specific definition, because it is difficult to measure its realisation in practice. This is a further conclusion based on the literature described in this report. It is also important for health care professionals to be aware of factors supporting and restricting patient's autonomy in order to be aware their own possibilities either to support (or restrict) the autonomy of other persons.

There is much literature in the area of autonomy, but the focus of studies varies and the groups under investigation are heterogenous. One of the focus groups in our project are elderly patients in health care organisations and nursing homes, because these patients are often dependent on health care professionals as their physical or mental condition inhibits independent living. Based on our overview, feeding of patients forms the largest area of research among nursing interventions, especially relating force-feeding. However, ethical concepts and many everyday nursing interventions have not been investigated at all, such as medication administration and taking care of patients' elimination and body hygiene, although these are interventions which are frequently carried out in nursing practice. Thus, there is a great need to study connections between nursing interventions and patient autonomy.

In the area of acute care, nursing research abounds. Especially studies connected with do-not-resuscitate-orders in the USA. There are also studies connected with the subject of euthanasia. There still seems to be the urgent need to study the ethics in acute settings in European countries, especially in connection with the use of technology and medical and nursing interventions. The same need can be identified in maternity and gynaecological care, even through the role of women as well as feminist ethics are being discussed .

The concept of privacy is also one the most fundamental concepts in health care and nursing ethics. It has been investigated especially in the 1960s and 1970s in the social sciences. In the area of health care, not many empirical studies can be found. In this concept lot of similarities can be found with the concept of autonomy. It too has no precise definition and it has many dimensions. The main dimensions described in this report are physical, informational, social and psychological ones (Burgoon 1982 ).

Empirical studies concerning the concept of privacy have mainly been connected with physical privacy, relating to the hospital environment, noise and space. Problems are concerned with the design of rooms, daily routines in the wards, and activities of health care professionals. There is a lack, however, regarding the knowledge about the conceptualisation of privacy as well as communication between nursing activities, privacy and well-being. In addition, information is another large area connected with privacy. It is connected with confidentiality of information in the health care system, with informatics and nurses' activities. This is an area, which needs further research. It is relevant to all areas of health care organisation.

The realisation of the concept of privacy is depending on both external and internal factors. Internal factors supporting privacy are described as behavioural mechanisms and external areas are divided into social relationships and physical environment. The internal factors restricting privacy include the sense of privacy and the external ones social relationships, regulation of information, physical boundaries, lack of physical space, and financial connections. There are problems with privacy in each of the patients' groups the present project is connected with. In the elderly, these are related to the environment of long-term wards. In acute care, the problems of privacy are physical, but also informational in nature. In maternity and gynaecological care, privacy has to do with the mother and baby, a highly sensitive relationship which calls for sensitivity on the part of professionals as well. There is a special need for privacy in gynaecological examinations and when using artificial reproductive technologies.

Informed consent is related to most activities in health care organisations. However, there is abundant literature concerning this concept. It is most often defined by using several elements. In this report, the concept of informed consent is divided into three dimensions. They are prerequisites, decision-making activities and outcomes. Empirical studies seem to concentrate on the dimensions of prerequisites and decision-making activities. The realisation of the informed consent is depending on several aspects, connected with the type of informed consent in question. The types are described using the dimensions of activity-passivity and explicit-implicit. The realisation of informed consent is connected with health care professionals and their different roles concerning the process of obtaining consent. For example, in many countries only physicians are allowed to inform patients about the diagnosis, and nurses can help the patients to know their rights and to act as patient advocates. Factors restricting informed consent include the competence of the patient, limited information, ineffective communication between patients and professionals, and hospital environment itself, and also problems of privacy.

Empirical studies related to informed consent are rather many. In part of these studies, the focus lies on hospital organisation in general and in the readability of the informed consent forms. Also, roles of different health care professionals and cultural differences have been under investigation. In the care of elderly, informed consent has been recently analysed by Sugarman et al (1998). In their review, understanding, recruitment and disclosure were the aspects mostly studied. In areas of acute care, informed consent has been studied especially in connection with surgical activities and anaesthesia. In maternity and gynaecological care, then, studies related to informed consent are rare and generally they are in the area of abortion and gynaecological examinations.

However, the biggest problem in the realisation of informed consent seems to be the information giving and the understanding of it. Here too are future research needs in Europe. It seems that professionals think they have given more information, than patients have understood. The problem can be in the content and language of information, or in the way of giving information – and this demands further studies. These studies are especially important for nurses, because they often have to explain details to patients, which have not been understood.

All the three concepts, autonomy, privacy and informed consent are close cousins that overlap, but there are certain differences. In addition, they are connected with the culture of each of the countries. Although the core of the concepts may be the same, the definitions of the concepts vary in different cultural areas, and also the importance of these concepts and their realisation. Also, the work of nurses has an international nature, and the ethical problems have a lot of similarities (e.g. Tadd 1998). In Europe, nursing education should follow the directives of the European Commission as it gives a basis for the homogenisation of using education. This needs emphasis in the teaching of ethics. Thus, in order to understand the differences between different countries, empirical work needs be done in future. Such work should be multi-professional, including not only health care organisations, but communities as a whole.

In general, we can conclude that the overview of the literature of the concepts autonomy, privacy, and informed consent has given some very clear indicators of a need for future research, which can be summarised as follows:

- Analysis of the realisation of the concepts of autonomy, privacy and informed consent in nursing and health care practice should be conducted. This means that more detailed conceptual definitions are needed. Also, the realisation of these concepts should be analysed in specific health care contexts. In nursing, it seems to be common, to describe the basic ethical principles on a theoretical level, but not in relation to specific practical contexts or nursing interventions. Deeper knowledge regarding the concepts presupposes concrete reflection of their application in practice.
- In-service education regarding the importance of the concepts and the impact such education has on the nurses' understanding of patients needs and consequently on more humane and effective nursing care.
- Teaching aspects related to the concepts in basic nursing courses as well as in post-graduate nursing programmes followed by evaluation research of their implementation.

# References

## Laws
*Finland*

The Act on the Amendment of the Act on the Status and Rights of Patients (333/98) Laki potilaan asemasta ja oikeuksista annetun lain muuttamisesta 15.5.1998. Helsinki: Suomen Säädöskokoelma.

The Act on the University of Helsinki Central Hospital (1064/89) Laki Helsingin yliopistollisesta keskussairaalasta 1.12.1989/1064. Helsinki: Suomen Säädöskokoelma.

The Act on Personal Data Register (471/87) Henkilörekisterilaki 30.4.1987/471. Helsinki: Suomen Säädöskokoelma.

The Act on the Status and Rights of Patients (785/92) Laki potilaan asemasta ja oikeuksista 17.8.1992/785. Helsinki: Suomen Säädöskokoelma.

The Act on Social Work with Intoxicant Abusers (41/86) Päihdehuoltolaki 17.1.1986/41. Helsinki: Suomen Säädöskokoelma.

The Act on Special Care for the Retarded (519/77) Laki kehitysvammaisten erityishuollosta 23.6.1977. Helsinki: Suomen Säädöskokoelma.

The Act Concerning Health Care Professionals (559/94) Laki terveydenhuollon ammattihenkilöistä 28.6.1994. Helsinki: Suomen Säädöskokoelma.

The Communicable Diseases Act (583/86) Tartuntatautilaki 25.7.1986. Helsinki: Suomen Säädöskokoelma.

The Constitutional Act (1919) Suomen Hallitusmuoto, Perustuslaki. 17.7.1919. Suomen Lakikirja.

The Decree on Personal Data Register (476/87) Henkilörekisteriasetus 30.4.1987. Helsinki: Suomen Säädöskokoelma.

The New Personal Data Act (532/99) Henkilötietolaki. 22.4.1999. Helsinki: Suomen Säädöskokoelma.

The Personal Data File Act (512/ 1986) Henkilörekisterilaki 19.6.1986. Helsinki: Suomen Säädöskokoelma.

The Act on the Interruption of Pregnancy (239/70) Laki raskauden keskeyttämisestä 24.3.1970. Helsinki: Suomen Säädöskokoelma.

The Act on National Personal Records Kept Under the Health Care System (556/89) Laki terveydenhuollon valtakunnallisista henkilörekistereistä 9.6.1989. Helsinki: Suomen Säädöskokoelma.

The Act on Primary Health Care (66/1972) Kansanterveyslaki 28.1.1972. Helsinki: Suomen Säädöskokoelma.

Act on the Removal of Human Organs and Tissues for Medical Use (355/1985) Laki ihmisen elimien ja kudosten irrottamisesta lääketieteelliseen käyttöön 26.4.1985. Helsinki: Suomen Säädöskokoelma.

The Act on Specialized Medical Care (1062/89) Erikoissairaanhoitolaki 1.12.1989. Helsinki: Suomen Säädöskokoelma.

The Castration Act (282/1970) Kastroimislaki 24.4.1970. Helsinki: Suomen Säädöskokoelma.

The Act on Sterilization (283/70) Steriloimislaki 24.4.1970. Helsinki: Suomen Säädöskokoelma.

The Decree on National Personal Records Kept Under the Helth System (774/89) Asetus terveydenhuollon valtakunnallisesta henkilörekisteristä 1.9.1989. Helsinki: Suomen Säädöskokoelma.

The Mental Health Act (1116/90) Mielenterveyslaki 14.12.1990. Helsinki: Suomen Säädöskokoelma.

The Occupational Health Care Act (743/78) Työterveyshuoltolaki. 29.9.1978. Helsinki: Suomen Säädöskokoelma.

The Patient Injury Act (585/86) Potilasvahinkolaki 25.7.1986. Helsinki: Suomen Säädöskokoelma.

The Private Health Care Act (1136/92) Laki yksityisestä terveydenhuollosta 27.11.92. Helsinki: Suomen Säädöskokoelma.

The Act on Public Documents (83/51) Laki yleisten asiakirjain julkisuudesta 9.2.1951. Helsinki: Suomen Säädöskokoelma.

*References*

*Germany*

The Constitution (1991) Grundgesetz. Die Verfassung von Berlin und das Grundgesetz für die
    Bundesrepublik Deutschland. Berlin: Landeszentrale für politische Bildungsarbeit.
Criminal Court Procedure (1998) Strafprozessordnung 29. Auflage. München: Beck-Texte in Deutscher
    Taschenbuchverlag.
Criminal Code (1999) Strafgesetzbuch. 33. Auflage. München: Deutscher Taschenbuchverlag.
Law of Social Care (1979) Heimgesetz. Gesetz über Altenheime, Altenwohnheime und Pflegeheime für
    Volljährige. 2. Auflage. München: Beck'sche Verlagsbuchhandlung.
Social Security Code (1990) Sozialgesetzbuch XI. Arbeits- und Sozialrecht der Bundesrepublik
    Deutschland. Auswahl aus der Sammlung: Das Deutsche Bundesrecht. Baden-Baden: Nomos
    Verlagsgesellschaft.
Civil Rights Court Procedure (1992) Zivilprozessordnung. 22. Auflage. München: C.H.Beck'sche
    Verlagsbuchhandlung.

*Greece*

Ministerial Circular (1990) Examination of HIV in Humans. No 4548. Athens: Ministry of Health.
Civil Code (1984) Presidential Degree No 456. Athens: Official Gazette.
Code on the Practice of Medicine (1939) No 1565. Athens: Official Gazette A 16.
Code of the House of Correction (1969) A.N. 125. Athens: Official Gazette.
Reform and Organization of Health System (1992) Law No 2071. Athens: Official Gazette.
Equality of Men and Women-Reform of Family Law (1983) Law No 1329. Athens: Official Gazette.
Ministerial Decision (1984) No A6 10983. Clinical Trials on Drugs. Athens: Official Gazette.
National Health System (1983) Law No 1397. Athens: Official Gazette.
Penal Code (1950) No 1492. Athens: Official Gazette.
Person's protection from personal data processing (1997) Law No 2472. Athens: Official Gazette.
Presidential Degree (1985) Penal Code No 283. Athens: Official Gazette.

*Spain*

Act (1979) 30/1979 del 27 de octubre. (BOE 6/11/79) Extracción y transplante de órganos.
Act (1988) 35/1988 del 22 de noviembre. (BOE 24/11/88) Técnicas de reproducción asistida.
Act (1990) 25/1990 del 20 de diciembre. (BOE 22/12/90). Ley del Medicamento.
Civil Code (1889) 24 julio 1889.
Decree (1996) 284/1996 del 23 de juliol.( DOG 31/7/96) Regulació del Sistema Català de Serveis Socials.
Order 1477 (1991) del 10 julio 1991.(D.O.G de 7/8/91). Acreditació de Centres Hospitalaris de Catalunya.
Organic Act (1982) 1/1982 del 5 de mayo.(BOE 14/5/82) De protección civil del derecho al honor, a la
    intimidad personal y familiar y a la propia imagen.
Organic Act (1992) 5/1992 del 29 de octubre. (BOE 31/10/92) Regulación del tratamiento automatizado
    de los datos de carácter personal (LORTRAD).
Penal Code (1995) 23 de Noviembre 1995.
The Spanish Constitution (1978) 27 de diciembre 1978. (BOE 29/12/78).
The General Health Act (1986) 14/1986 de 25 de Abril. (BOE 29/4/86).
The Royal Decree (1978) 2082/1978 de 28 de Agosto. (Abolished).
The Royal Decree (1978) 944/1978 del 14 de abril. (Abolished).
The Royal Decree (1980) 426/1980 del 22 de febrero. (BOE 13/4/80). Extracción y Transplantes de
    Organos.
The Royal Decree (193) 561/1993 del 16 de abril. (BOE 13/5/93). Requisitos para la realización de
    ensayos clínicos con medicamentos.

*The United Kingdom*

Abortion Act (1967) London: HMSO.
Access to Health Records Act (1990 - English) London: HMSO.
Access to Health Records (1991) (Steps to secure compliance and complaints procedures Scotland Regulations). Scottish office, NHS in Scotland Management Executive. Edinburgh: HMSO.
Access Modification Act (Health) Order (1987) London: HMSO.
The Age of Legal Capacity (Scotland) Act (1991) London: HMSO.
The Childrens Act (1989) London: HMSO.
Computer Misuse Act (1990) London: HMSO.
Data Protection Act (1984) London: HMSO.
Data Protection Act (1998) London: HMSO.
Family Law Reform Act (1969) London: HMSO.
Human Fertilisation and Embryo Act (1990) London: HMSO.
Mental Health (Scotland) Act (1960) Edinburgh: HMSO.
Mental Health (Northern Ireland) Order (1986) Belfast: HMSO.
Mental Health (England and Wales) Act (1983)London: HMSO.
Mental Health (Scotland) Act (1984) Edinburgh: HMSO.
Mental Health Patients in the Community Act (1995) London: HMSO.
Nurses, Midwives and Health Visitors Acts (1979) London: HMSO.
Nurses, Midwives and Health Visitors Acts (1992)London: HMSO.
The Patients Charter (1991) Department of Health. London: HMSO.


**Codes of Ethics**

Automatic Processing of Personal Data (1981) European Treaty Series No. 108. European Commission.
Code of Ethics of the International Association of Medical Laboratory Technologists (1992) IAMLT. Dublin 29 July, 1992.
Convention for Protection of Human Rights and Dignity of the Human Being with Regard to the Application of Biology and Medicine: Convention on Human Rights and Biomedicine (1997) Onedo, 4.IV, European Treaty Series. European Commission.
Convention for Protection of Human Rights and Fundamental Freedoms (1950) Council of Europe, European Treaties, ETS No 5. Rome 4.XI.1950. Amended by Protocol No. 11 (ETS) No. 155 of May, 1994. Council of Europe. European Treaties. European Commission.
Declaration of Children's Rights (1989) Lapsen oikeuksia koskeva yleissopimus. Hyväksytty 20.3.1989, New York. Lapsen oikeuksia koskevan yleissopimuksen voimaansaattamisesta sekä yleissopimuksen eräiden määräysten hyväksymisestä annetun lain voimaantulosta 16.8.1991/1130. SopS:60/1991. Sosiaali- ja terveydenhuoltolainsäädäntö. Lakimiesliiton Kustannus. Helsinki: Kauppakaari Oy, 293-301.
Declaration of Euthanasia (1987) Adopted by the 39th World Medical Assembly, Madrid, Spain, October 1987. In Lääkärin etiikka (1996) Suomen Lääkäriliitto. Forssa: Forssan Kirjapaino Oy, 119.
Declaration of Geneva (1968) Adopted by the 2nd WMA General Assembly, Geneva, Switzerland, September 1948 and amended by the 22 nd World Medical Asssembly, Sidney, Australia, August 1968 and the 35 th World Medical Assembly, Venice, Italy, October 1983 and the 46th WMA General Assembly, Stockholm, Sweden, September 1994. In Lääkärin etiikka (1996). Suomen Lääkäriliitto. Forssa: Forssan Kirjapaino Oy, 113.
Declaration of Helsinki (1964) Adopted by the 18th World Medical Assembly, Helsinki, Finland, June 1964, amended by the 29th World Medical Assembly, Tokyo, Japan, October 1975, the 35th World Medical Asssembly, Venice, Italy, October 1983, and the 41st World Medical Assembly, Hong Kong, September 1989. In Lääkärin etiikka (1996). Suomen Lääkäriliitto. Forssa: Forssan Kirjapaino Oy, 114-11 6.
Declaration of Lisbon (1981, 1993) Adopted by the 34th World Medical Assembly, Lisbon, Portugal,

September/October 1981 and amended by the 47th General Assembly, Bali, Indonesia, September 1995. Suomen Lääkärilehti 32, 3498-3499.

Declaration of Oslo (1970) Statement on Therapeutic Abortion. Adopted by the 24th World Medical Assembly, Oslo, Norway, August 1970, and amended by the 35th World Medical Assembly, Venice, Italy, October 1983. In Lääkärin etiikka (1992) Suomen Lääkäriliitto. Forssa: Forssan Kirjapaino, 94.

Declaration of Promotion of Patients' Rights in Europa (1994) A WHO European Consultation on the Rights of Patients, meeting in Amsterdam 28-30 March, 1994. WHO Regional Office for Europe.

Declaration of Sidney (1968) Statement of Death. Adopted by the 22nd World Medical Assembly, Sidney, Australia, August 1968, and amended by the 35th World Medical Assembly, Venice, Italy, October 1983. In Lääkärin Etiikka (1992) Suomen Lääkäriliitto. Forssa: Forssan Kirjapaino Oy, 93-94.

Declaration of Tokyo (1975) Adopted by the 29th World Medical Assembly, Tokyo, Japan, October 1975.

European Social Charter (1961) Turin, 18.X.1961. Concil of Europe, European Treaties.

The International Codes of Medical Ethics (1983) Adopted by the 3rd General Assembly of the World Medical Association, London England, October 1949, amended by the 22nd World Medical Assembly, Sidney, Australia, August 1968, and the 35th World Medical Assembly, Venice, Italy, October 1983. In Lääkärin Etiikka (1992) Suomen Lääkäriliitto. Forssa: Forssan Kirjapaino Oy, 84-85.

ICN (1973) International Council of Nurses: Code for Nurses.

International Covenant on Civil and Political Rights (1966) The United Nations General Assembly Resolution 2200 A(XXI) of 16, December 1996.

The Nüremberg Code (1949) In E.L. Bandman & B. Bandman. Nursing ethics through the life span. (2nd ed.). Appleton & Lange, Norwalk, CT.

International Covenant on Economic, Social and Cultural Rights (1976) U.N.T.S. No 14531 Vol 993, 3.

Twelve Principles of Provisions of Health Care in Any Natural Health Care System (1963)

The Universal Declaration of Human Rights (1948) Copenhagen: United Nations Information Centre, UNIC.


**Professional Codes**

American Nurses Association (1976) Code for Nurses. With Interpretative Statements. Kansas City, MO: American Nurses' Association.

IAMLT (1992) Code of Ethics of International Association of Medical Laboratory Technologists. 29.7.1992, Dublin.

International Council of Nurses (1973) Code for Nurses Ethical Concepts Applied to Nursing. ICN, Geneva, Switzerland.

International Confederation of Midwives (1993) International Code of Ethics for Midwive. Adopted by the International Confederation of Midwives Council, Vancouver, May, 1993. Registered Charity No. 326297.

Principles of the European Medical Deontology (1987) Standing Committee of Doctors of the European Community. Brussels.


*Finland*

Finnish Association of Physiotherapists (1998) Suomen Fysioterapeuttiliitto. Fysioterapeutin eettiset periaatteet. Suomen Fysioterapeuttiliitto.

Suomen Röntgenhoitajaliitto (1992) Röntgenhoitajan eettiset periaatteet. Suomen Röntgenhoitajaliitty ry.

Suomen Lastenhoitoalan liitto (1993) Lastenhoidon eettiset periaatteet. Suomen lastenhoitoalan liitto ry.

Finnish Federation of Mental Health Nurses (1997) Suomen Mielenterveyshoitajaliiton eettiset periaatteet.

Suomen Mielenterveyshoitajaliitto.
Finnish Society of Intensive Care (1997) Suomen Tehohoitoyhdistys. Suomen Tehohoitoyhdistyksen eettiset ohjeet. STHY. Suomen Tehohoitoyhdistys.
The Finnish Union of Practical Nurses (1996) Super. Lähihoitajan eettiset ohjeet. Suomen lähi- ja perushoitajaliitto. Offset-Koppinen.
Tehy (1997) Ethical Guidelines of Nurses. Sairaanhoitaja 70 (7), 43.


*Germany*


Anonymous (1995) Wittenberger Thesen - Vorschläge zum ersten Kontakt mit der Psychiatrie. Psychosoziale Umschau (3), 23-24.
Arbeitsgemeinschaft katholischer Pflegeorganisationen (1995) Die ethische Verantwortung der Pflegeberufe 9-13, Mainz: AKP.
Caritas Gemeinschaft für Pflege und Sozialberufe e.V; Deutscher Caritas Verband e.V., and Katholischer Berufsverband für Pflegeberufe e.V. (1998) Die ethische Verantwortung der Pflegeberufe. Freiburg: Deutscher Caritas Verband.
Caritas Schwesternschaft e.V. (1987) Ethik im Pflegealltag. Zwangslage der Moral für Krankenschwestern und -pfleger in einer sich verändernden Gesellschaft. (Irish Guid of Catholic Nurses: Moral Dilemmas for Nurses in a changing society. Translated by Marianne Arndt), Freiburg: Caritas-Gemeinschafte.V. Freiburg.
Behindertenhilfe (1995) Ethische Grundaussagen der vier Fachverbände der Behindertenhilfe. Ethik in der Medizin, 154-155.
Deutscher Berufsverband für Pflegeberufe e.V. (1992) Berufsordnung des DBfK. Eschborn: DBfK Verlag.
Deutscher Berufsverband für Pflegeberufe e.V. (1995) Die Herausforderung Gesundheit 2000 - Implikationen für die Pflegeberufe. In Gesundheitswesen 2000, Edited by: DBfK, Eschborn: DBfK Verlag.
Evangelischer Fachverband für Kranken und Sozialpflege (1993/94) Ethische Leitlinien. Frankfurt: Mitteilungen des Ev. Fachverbandes für Kranken- und Sozialpflege e.V.
International Council of Nursing (1973) Ethische Grundregeln für die Krankenpflege. Frankfurt/Genf: ICN.
Schwesternschaft des Ev. Diakonievereins e.V. (1996) Pflege- und Dienstverständnis der Schwestern im Ev. Diakonieverein. Berlin: Schwesternschaft des Ev. Diakonievereins e.V.
Verband der Schwesternschaften vom Deutschen Roten Kreuz (1995) Berufsethische Grundsätze der Schwesternschaften vom Deutschen Roten Kreuz. Bonn: DRK.


*Greece*


Athens Medical Association (1984) European Map of the Rights of Patients. AMA News Letter 29, 21-31.
Nursing Code of Ethics (1996) Nossileftiki 1 (35), 2-6.


*Spain*


Ethical Code of Nursing (1986) Código de Ética de Enfermería. Col.legit Diplomats d'Infermeria de Barcelona. Catalonia.
Deontological Code of the Spanish Nursing (1989) Código Deontológico de la Enfermería Española. Madrid: General Council of Nurses Spain.
Guidelines about Informed Consent (1997) Guia de recomanacions sobre el Consentiment Informat. Barcelona, Spain: Generalitat de Catalunya.
A Practical guide to Informed Consent (1997) Guia Práctica Consentimiento Informado. Spain: Comunidad Foral de Navarra Pamplona.

Patient's rights bill of the hospital (1984) (Drets del malalt/usuari d'Hospital) Departament de Sanitat i
    Seguretat Social. Generalitat de Catalunya.


*The United Kingdom*

Anonymous Testing for the Prevalence of the Human Immune Deficiency Virus (HIV) (1994) London:
    UKCC.
Confidentiality: use of computers, position statement (1992) London: UKCC.
Complementary Therapies, position statement (1995) London: UKCC.
Guidelines for Professional Practice (1996) London: UKCC.
Midwives Rules (1993) London: UKCC.
The Midwives Code of Practice (1994) London: UKCC.
The Scope of Professional Practice (1992) London: UKCC.
Standards for the Administration of Medicines (1992) London: UKCC.
Standards for Records and Record Keeping (1993) London: UKCC.
UKCC (1992) Code of professional conduct for the nurse, midwife and health visitor. London: UKCC.
UKCC (1996) Guidelines for Professional Practice. London: UKCC.


**Other references**

Abades, M. & Gasull, M. (1995) Principis ètics i escales de medició del grau d'autonomia i dependència de
    les persones ancianes. 4th Simposi d'Atenció Sòcio-Sanitària.Ponèncias i Comunicaciones.
    Barcelona: Generalitat de Catalunya.
Abel, F. (1990) Dinamismo del diálogo bioético en una España en transición. Boletin Oficial Sanitario
    Panamericano 108 (5-6), 542-549.
Abraham I., Chalifoux Z., Evers G. & de Geest S. (1995) Conditions, interventions, and outcomes in
    nursing research: a comparative analysis of North American and European International
    journals (1981-1990). International Journal of Nursing Studies 32, 173-187.
Abrams, N. (1978) A contrary view of the nurse as patient advocate. Nursing Forum 17 (3), 258-267.
Aiken, T.D. & Catalano, J.T. (1994) Legal, ethical and political issues in nursing. Philadelphia: F.A. Davis
    Company.
Allekian, C. (1973) Intrusions of territory and personal space: an anxiety-inducing factor for hospitalized
    persons - an exploratory study. Nursing Research 22 (3), 236-241.
Allekian, C. (1974) Intrusions of territory and personal space: an exploratory study of anxiety-inducing
    factors in hospitalised patients. The International Journal of Psychiatry of Medicine 5 (1), 27-39.
Allison, C., Page, H. & George, S. (1994) Screening for coronary heart disease risk factors in retail
    pharmacies in Sheffield. Journal of Epidemiology and Community Health 48 (2), 178-181.
Altman, I. (1975) The environment and social behavior. Privacy, personal space, territory, crowding.
    Monterey: Cole Publishing Company.
Altman, I. (1976) Privacy: a conceptual analysis. Environment and Behavior 8 (1), 7-29.
Altman, I. (1977) Privacy regulation: culturally universal or culturally specific? Journal of Social Issues 33
    (3), 66-84.
Altman, I. & Vinsel, A. (1977) Personal space. An analysis of E.T. Hall's proxemics framework. In I.
    Altman & J. Wohlwill (eds.) Human behavior and environment. Advances in theory and
    research, Vol 2. New York: Plenum Press, 181-259.
Altmann, B. & Münch, K. (1997) Meinen Körper kenne ich selbst am besten. Eine Studie zur
    Selbstbestimmung in Pflegesituationen aus Sicht von Patienten. Diplomarbeit (Pflegepädagogik)
    128/97. Humboldt Universität, Berlin.
Amelung, E. (Ed.) (1992) Ethisches Denken in der Medizin. Germany.
Amstrong-Esther, C., Sandilands, M. & Miller, D. (1989) Attitudes and behaviours of nurses towards the
    elderly in an acute care setting. Journal of Advanced Nursing 14, 34-44.

Amstrong-Esther, C., Browne, K. & McAfee, J. (1994) Elderely patients: still clean and sitting quietly. Journal of Advanced Nursing 19, 264-271.

Annas, G. (1981) Invasion of privacy in the hospital. Nursing Law and Ethics 2 (1), 3.

Anapliotou-Vazaiou, I. (1993) General principles of medical law. Athens: Sakkoula.

Androulaki-Dimitriadi, I. (1993) The obligation of patient's information. Athens: Sakkoula.

Anrys, H. (1998) Medical ethics and human rights. In The human rights, ethical and moral dimensions of health care. European Network of Scientific Co-operation on Medicine and Human Rights. Germany: Council of Europe Publishing, 55-58.

Antón, P. (1984) Enfermeria etíca y legislacion. Ediciones cientificas y tecnicas. Barcelona: Masson-Salvat.

van der Arend, A. & Gastmans, C. (1996) Ethik für Pflegende. Bern: Hans Huber Verlag.

Arndt, M. (1994) Nurses' medication errors: an interpretive study of experiences. Frankfurt: Peter Lang.

Arndt, M. (1996a) Ethik denken - Maßstäbe zum Handeln in der Pflege. Stuttgart: Georg Thieme Verlag.

Arndt, M. (1996b) Spannungsfeld Arbeitsauftrag und Medizinische Ethik: Die Pflegeberufe in der invasiven operativen Krankenhausroutine. Die Schwester/Der Pfleger 35 (1), 7-16.

Arndt, M. (1997a) Vermittlung von Diagnose und Prognose-die Rolle der Pflegenden. Forum 12 (2), 123-127.

Arndt, M. (1997b) Nicht frei zum Moralischen Handeln. Die Schwester/Der Pflege 36 (6), 516-521.

Arndt, M. (1998a) Werte in der pflegerischen Wirklichkeit. Die Schwester/Der Pfleger 37 (5), 435-441.

Arndt, M. (1998b) How can nurses and midwives confront the challanges of global evolution and improve the quality of life? CICAMS News, 3rd and 4th Trimester, 19-23.

Athlin, L., Engström, B. & Engström, I. (1992) Information to patients following surgery for cancer. [Information till patienter efter operation för cancersjukdom.]Vård i Norden 12 (1), 4-7.

Bailey, R.N. (1994) The doctor-patient relationship: communication, informed consent and the optometric patient. Journal of the American Optometric Association 65 (6), 418-422.

Balaskas, J. & Gordon, J. (1989) The encyclopedia of pregnancy and birth. London: MacDonald & Co.

Ballou, K. (1998) A concept analysis of autonomy. Journal of Professional Nursing 14 (2), 102-110.

Bandman, E.L. & Bandman, B. (1995) Nursing ethics through the life span. (3rd ed.). Norwalk, CT: Appleton & Lange.

Barbero, J. (1996) Problemas éticos en la atención al anciano enfermo. Labor Hospitalaria 243, 53-64.

Barclay, C. (1998) Intimate examinations without tears. Trends in Urology, Gynaecoloogy and Sexual Health 3, 25-28.

Bard, T.R. (1990) Medical ethics in practice. Washington: Hemisphere Publishing Corporation.

Barnes, D.M., Davis, A.J., Moran, T., Portillo, C.J. & Koenig, B.A. (1998) Informed consent in a multicultural cancer patient population: implications for nursing practice. Nursing Ethics 5 (5), 412-423.

Barnett, K. (1972) A survey of the current utilization of touch by health team personnel with hospitalized patients. International Journal of Nursing Studies 9, 195-209.

Barron, A. (1990) The right to personal life. Nursing Times 86 (27), 28-32.

Bauer, I. (1994) Patients' privacy: exploratory study of patients' perceptions of their privacy in a German acute care hospital. Developments in Nursing and Health Care 3. Aldershot: Avebury Ashgate.

Beardsley, E. (1971) Privacy: autonomy and selective disclosure. In J. Pennock & J. Chapman (eds.) Privacy. New York: Atherton Press, 56-70.

Beardsley, R., Johnson, C. & Benson, S. (1977) Privacy as a factor in patient counselling. Journal of the American Pharmacentical Association 17 (6), 366-368.

Beauchamp, T.L. & Childress, J.F. (1994) Principles of biomedical ethics (4th ed.). New York: Oxford University Press.

Benfield, D., Flaksman, R., Lin, T.H., Kantak, A., Kokomoor, F. & Vollman, J. (1991) Teaching intubation skills using newly deceased infants. Journal of American Medical Association 265 (18), 2360-2363.

Benn, S. (1971) Privacy, freedom, and respect for persons. In J. Pennock & J. Chapman (eds.) Privacy. New York: Atherton Press, 1-26.

Bergman, R. & Goldander, H. (1982) Evaluation of care for the aged: a multipurpose guide. Journal of

Advanced Nursing 7, 203-207.

Besch, L. (1979) Informed consent: a patient's right. Nursing Outlook 27 (1), 32-35.

Bexell, G., Norberg, A. & Norberg, B. (1985) Ethical conflicts in long-term care of aged patients. An ontological model of the care situation. Ethics and Medicine 1 (3), 44-46.

Biley, F. (1992) Some determinants that affect patient participation in decision-making about nursing care. Journal of Advanced Nursing 17, 414-421.

Blackhall, L.J., Murphy, S.T., Frank, G., Michel, V. & Azen, S. (1995) Ethnicity and attitudes toward patient autonomy. The Journal of the American Medical Association 274 (24), 820-825.

Blanchard, C., Ruckdeschel, J., Fletcher, B. & Blanchard, E. (1986) The impact of oncologists' behaviors on patient satisfaction with morning rounds. Cancer 58 (2), 387-393.

Bobak, I., Jensen, M. & Zalar, M. (1989) Maternity and gynaegological care. The nurse and the family. St Louis: C.V. Mosby.

Bockenheimer-Lucius, G. (1995) Die Bioethik-Konvention. Ethik in der Medizin 7(3), 146-153.

Boladeras, M. (1998) Bioética. Madrid: Síntesis.

Bolam v Friern Hospital Management Committee (1957) All England Law Report 2.

Bond, S. & Thomas, L. (1992) Measuring patients' satisfaction with nursing care. Journal of Advanced Nursing 17, 52-63.

Bouchard, L. (1993) Patients' satisfaction with the physical environment of an oncology clinic. Journal of Psychosocial Oncology 11 (1), 55-67.

Boucher, M. (1971) Personal space and chronicity in the mental hospital. Perspectives in Psychiatric Care 9 (5), 206-210.

Bradley, A.W. & Ewing, K.D. (1997) Constitutional and administrative law (12th ed.). Essex: Addison Wesley Longman.

Branningan, V. & Beier, B. (1995) Patient privacy in the era of medical computer networks: a new paradigm or a new technology. Medinfo 8 Pt 1, 640-643.

Brazier, M. (1987) Medicine, patients and the law. Middlesex: Penguin Books.

Brazier, M. & Lobjoit, M. (1991) Protecting the vulnerable. Autonomy and consent in health care. London: Routledge.

Brennan, M, (1997) A concept analysis of consent. Journal of Advanced Nursing 25, 477-484.

Brenner, G. (1997) Rechtskunde für das Krankenpflegepersonal einschliesslich des Altenpflegepersonals und anderer Berufe im Gesundheitswesen. Stuttgart: Fischer Verlag.

British Medical Association (1995) Medical ethics today: its practice and philosophy. Reprinted. BMJ Publishing Group. Plymouth: Latimer Trend & Company.

Brody, D.S. (1980) The patient's role in clinical decision-making. Annals of Internal Medicine 93, 718-22.

Broggi, M.A. (1995) La información clínica y el consentimiento informado. Problemas en la aplicación del consentimiento informado. Medicina Clínica 104 (6), 24-26.

Broggi, M.A. (1998a) Cultural differences in the process of information giving and patient consent. EDTNA/ERCA (European Dialysis and Transplant Nurses Association and European Renal Care Association.) In press.

Broggi, M.A. (1998b) La Bioética como ayuda clínica. La Gestión Hospitalaria. Barcelona: Masson Ed.

Brown, J.M., Kitson, A.L., & McKnight, T.J. (1992) Challenges in caring: explorations in nursing and ethics. London: Chapman and Hall.

Buchanan, M. (1995) Enabling patients to make informed decisions. Nursing Times 91 (18), 27-29.

Bulechek, G.M. & McCloskey J.C. (1992) Defining and validating nursing interventions. Nursing Clinincs of North America 27 (2), 289-299.

Burden, B. (1998) Privacy or help? The use of curtain positioning strategies within the maternity ward environment as a means of achieving and maintaining privacy, or as a form of signalling to peers and professionals in an attempt to seek information and support. Journal of Advanced Nursing 27, 15-23.

Burgess, C., Davies, S. & Own, M. (1988) The way forward. Nursing the Elderly 1 (2), 19-21.

Burgoon, J. (1982) Privacy and communication. Communication Yearbook 6, 206-249.

Burt, R.A. (1996) The supressed legacy of Nuremberg. Hastings Center Report 26 (5), 30-33.

Byrne, D.J., Napier, A. & Cushieri, A. (1988) How informed is signed consent? British Medical Journal

269 (19), 839-840.

Bäck, E. & Wikblad, K. (1998) Privacy in hospital. Journal of Advanced Nursing 27 (5), 940-945.

Böhme, H. (1991) Das Recht des Krankenpflegepersonals, Teil 2 (3. Auflage). Stuttgart: Kohlhammer Verlag.

Cahill, J. (1994) Are you prepared to be their advocate? Issues in patient advocacy. Professional Nurse 9 (6), 371-372, 374-375.

De la Calle, A., Fernandez-Miranda, C., Moreno, E., Dongil, M. & Trueba, J.L. (1999) Consentimiento informado. Comunicación e información oral y escrita en 935 pacientes quirúrgicos. II Congreso Nacional. Asociación de Bioética Fundamental y Clínica. Madrid.

Calkins, M. (1995) Home-like, it's more than carpeting and chintz. Nursing Homes 44 (6), 20-25.

Callens, S. (1993) The automatic processing of medical data in Belgium: is the individual protected? Medical Law 12, 55-59.

Campbell, J. (1984) Anxiety and satisfaction of patients in four hospital designs. Dissertation Abstracts International 46, 112-b. (University Microfilms No 8504987).

Camps, V. (1999) Moral Pública y Moral Privada. II Congreso National. Asociación de Bioética fundamental y Clínica. Madrid.

Cantrell, T. (1978) Privacy - the medical problems. In J. Younger (ed.) Privacy. Chichester: John Wiley & Sons, 195-214.

Carey, M. & Helander, P. (1993) Hoitokäytäntöjen ja -ympäristön yhteys itsemääräämisoikeuden toteutumiseen synnyttäjien arvioimana. Pro gradu-tutkielma, Kuopion yliopisto. Kuopio: Yhteiskuntatieteellinen tiedekunta.

Canterbury v Spence (1972) 464 F 2d 772 DC, 1972.

Carpenito, L. (1989) Developments in nursing classification. In American Nurses Association, classification systems for describing nursing practice. Washington: American Nurses Publishing, 13-19.

Cassileth, B.R., Zupkis, R.V., Sutton-Smith, K. & March, V. (1980) Information and participation preferences among cancer patients. Annals of Internal Medicine 92 (6), 832-836.

Castellucci, D.T. (1998) Issues for nurses regarding elder autonomy. Nursing Clinics of North America 33 (2), 265-274.

Catlin, A.J. (1998) When pregnant women and their physicians disagree on the need for Cesarean section: no simple solution. Advanced Practice Nursing Quarterly 4 (2), 23-29.

Chadwick, R & Tadd, W. (1992) Ethics and nursing practice. Basingstone: Macmillan Press.

Chatterton v Gerson (1981) 1 All ER 245.

Chervenak, F.A. & McCullough, L. (1992) Ethical issues in obstetric ultrasonography. Clinical Obstetric and Gynecology 35 (4), 758-762.

Chervenak, F.A. & McCullough, L. (1993a) The importance of ethics to the practice of obstetric ultrasound. Annals of Medicine 25, 271-273.

Chervenak, F.A. & McCullough, L. (1993b) Identifying and managing ethical conflicts in the gynecologist-patient relationship. Journal of Reproductive Medicine 38 (7), 553-557.

Chervenak, F.A. & McCullough, L.B (1997) Ethics in obstetrics and gynecology. An overview. European Journal of Obstetrics, Gynecology and Reproductive Biology 75 (1), 91-94.

Chervenak, F.A. & McCullough, L.B. (1998a) Ethical issues in gynecology. Ceska Gynekologie 63 (2), 103-107.

Chervenak, F.A. & McCullough, L.B. (1998b) Ethical dimensions of ultrasound screening for fetal anomalies. Annals of the New York Academy of Sciences 18, 185-190.

Chipeur, G. (1993) Blood testing without consent: the right to privacy versus the right to know (Part I). Medicine and Law 12, 521-533.

Chou, D. (1996) Internet: road to heaven or hell for the clinical laboratory? Clinical Chemistry 42 (5), 827-830.

Clark, S., Leighton, B. & Seltzer, J. (1991) A risk-specific anesthesia consent form may hinder the infromed consent process. Journal of Clinical Anesthesia 3 (1), 11-13.

Clark, J. & Lang, N. (1992) Nursing's next advance: an international classification for nursing practice. International Nursing Review 39 (4), 109-111, 128.

Cobo, N., Nogueira, R. & Accala, J. (1999) Opinion de los usuarios sobre el consentimiento infarmado en una unidad de cuidadod intensivos. II Congreso National. Asociación de Bioética Fundamental y Clínica. Madrid.

Cohen, L.M., McCue, J.D. & Green, G.M. (1993) Do clinical and formal assessments of the capacity of patients in the intensive care unit to make decisions agree? Archives of Internal Medicine 153 (8), 2481-2485.

Colette, J. (1984) Role demands, privacy and psychological well-being. The International Journal of Socialpsychiatry 30 (3), 222-230.

Collopy, B. (1988) Autonomy in long-term care: some crucial distinctions. Gerontologist 28 (suppl), 10-17.

Collopy, B., Boyle, P. & Jennings, B. (1991) Conflicts in ethics. New directions in nursing home ethics. Geriatric Nursing 12 (4), 197-198.

Cooper, K. (1984) Territorial behavior among the institutionalized. A nursing perspective. Journal of Psychosocial Nursing 22 (12), 6-11.

Cooper, E. (1991) Balancing the scales of public interest: medical research and privacy. The Medical Journal of Australia 155, 556-560.

Corbella, J. (1996) El Dret a la protecció de la intimitat del malalt. Límits dels informes mèdics. Conference in Mestratge d'Especialització Mèdica. Unpublished.

Cortina, A., Arroyo, P., Torralba, M.J. & Zagusti, J. (1996) Ética y legislación en Enfermería Madrid: McGraw-Hill Interamericana.

Council of Europe (1996) Nursing research, report and recommendations. Strasbourg.

Crafter, H. & Rowan, C. (1998) Ethical issues in maternity care. In W. Tadd (ed.) Ethical issues in nursing and midwifery practice. Prespectives from Europe. Hampshire: McMillan, 103-123.

Cross, A.W. & Churchill, L.R. (1982) Ethical and cultural dimensions of informed consent. Annals of Internal Medicine 96, 110-113.

Crowe, B. & McDonald, I. (1997) Telemedicine in Australia. Recent development. Journal Telemed Telecare 3 (4), 188-193.

Cunningham, J. (1989) "What have I done? The issue of informed consent. Rehabilitation Nursing 14 (4), 202-203.

Curtin, L. (1981) Privacy: belonging to oneself. Perspectives in Psychiatric Care 19 (3-4), 112-115.

Cüer, P. (1998) Initiation to bioethics. In The human rights, ethical and moral dimensions of health care. European Network of Scientific Co-operation on Medicine and Human Rights. Council of Europe Publishing, Germany, 23-37.

Dal-Ré, R. (1992) Elements of informed consent in clinical research with drugs: a survey of Spanish clinical investigators. Journal of Internal Medicine 231, 375-379.

Dalla-Vorgia, P., Katsouyanni, K., Garanis, T., Touloumi, G., Drogaru, P. & Koutselinis, A. (1992) Attitudes of a Medditerranean population to the truth-telling issue. Journal of Medical Ethics 18, 67-74.

Davies, A. (1983) Ethical dilemmas and nursing practice. East Nortwalk: Prentice-Hall, Inc.

Davies, S., Laker, S. & Ellis, L. (1997) Promoting autonomy and independence for older people within nursing practice: a literature review. Journal of Advanced Nursing 26 (2), 408-417.

Davies, A. & Peters, M. (1983) Stresses of hospitalization in the elderly: nurses' and patients' perceptions. Journal of Advanced Nursing 8, 99-105.

Davies, A. & Snaith, P. (1980) The social behaviour of geriatric patients at mealtimes: an observational and an intervention study. Age and Aging 9, 93-99.

Davis, A. (1988) The clinical nurse's role in informed consent. Journal of Professional Nursing 4, 88-91.

Davis, A.J. (1989) Clinical nurses' ethical decision making in situations of informed consent. Advances in Nursing Science 11 (3), 63-69.

Davis, J. (1984) Don't fence me in. American Journal of Nursing 84 (9), 1141-11443.

Davis, A. & Underwood, P. (1989) The competency quagmire: clarification of the nursing perspective concerning the issues of competence and informed consent. International Journal of Nursing Studies 26, 271-279.

Dawes, P.J.D., O'Keefe, L. & Adcock, S. (1992) Informed consent: the assessment of two structured interview approaches compared to the current approach. The Journal of Laryngology and Otology 106 (5), 420-424.

Day, L., Drought, T. & Davis, A.J. (1995) Principle-based ethics and nurses' attitudes towards artificial feeding. Journal of Advanced Nursing 21 (2), 295-298.

DeLong, A. (1970) The micro-spatial structure of the older person: some implications of planning the social and spatial environments. In L. Pastalan & D. Carson (eds.) Spatial behavior of older people. University of Michigan, Ann Arbor, 83-85.

Deftos, L. (1998) The evolving duty to disclosure the presence of genetic disease to relatives. Academic Medicine 73 (9), 962-968.

De la Calle, A., Fernandez-Miranda, C., Moreno, E., Dongil, M. & Trueba, J.L. (1999) Consentimiento informado. Comunicacíon e información oral y escrita en 935 pacientes quirúrgicos. II Congreso Nacional. Asociacíon de Bioética Fundamental y Clínica.Madrid.

Delgado, J.C. (1996) Del Maternalismo a la autonomía. Una transformación ética de la Enfermería. Centro de Salud 9 (1), 499-504.

Deloughery, G.L. (Ed.) (1995) Issues and trends in nursing (2nd ed.). St Louis: Mosby-Year Book, Inc.

Department of Health (1993) Changing childbirth. Part 1. Report of the Expert Maternity Group. London: HMSO.

Department of Health and Welsh Office (1994) Code of Practice: Mental Health Act, 1983. London: HMSO.

DeVille, K.A. & Kopelman, L.M. (1998) Moral and social issues regarding pregnant women who use and abuse drugs. Obstetrics and Gynecology Clinics of North America 25 (1), 237-254.

Dickenson, D. (1994) The right to know and the right to privacy: confidentiality, HIV and health care professionals. Nursing Ethics 1, 111-115.

Dierks, C. (1993) Medical confidentiality and data protection as influenced by modern technology. Medicine and Law 12, 547-551.

Dijkstra, A. (1998) Care dependency. An assessment instrument for use in long-term care facilities. Groningen: Stichting Drukkerij C., Regenboog.

Dimond, B. (1995). Legal aspects of nursing (2nd ed.). London: Prentice-Hall, International Ltd.

Dixon, E. & Park, R. (1990) Do patients understand written health information? Nursing Outlook 38, 278-281.

Donnelly, M.B.& Anderson, R.M. (1990) The role related attitudes of physicians, nurses, and dieticians in the treatment of diabetes. Medical Care 28 (2), 175-179.

Doukas, D.J. & McCullough, L.B. (1991) The values history. The evaluation of the patient's values and advance directives. The Journal of Family Practice 32 (2), 145-153.

Doyal, L. (1997) Human need and the right of patients to privacy. Journal of Contemporary Health Law and Policy 14, 1-21

Downie, R.S. & Calman, K.C. (1994) Healthy respect: ethics in health care. (2nd ed.). Oxford: Oxford Medical Publications.

Draper, H. (1998) Sterilization abuse. Women and consent to treatment. In M. Brazier & M. Lobjoit (eds.) Protecting the vulnerable. Autonomy and consent in health care. London: Routledge, 77-100.

Drew, C., Salmon, P. & Webb, L. (1989) Mothers', midwives' and obstetricians' views on the features of obstetric care with influence satisfaction with childbirth. British Journal of Obstetrics and Gynaecology 96, 1084-1088.

Dupuis, H. (1987) Ethical aspects of reproductive medicine. In S. Doxiadis (ed.) Ethical dilemmas in health promotion. Chichester: John Wiley & Sons, 147-156.

Dyer, A.R. & Bloch, S. (1987) Informed consent and psychiatric patient. Journal of Medical Ethics 13 (1), 12-16.

Dworkin, G. (1988). The theory and practice of autonomy. Cambridge: Cambridge University Press.

Eddington, C., Piper, J., Tanna, B., Hodkinson, H. & Salmon, P. (1990) Relationships between happiness, behavioural status and dependencey on others in elderly patients. British Journal of Clinical Psychology 29, 43-50.

Edgar, A. (1994) Confidentiality and personal integrity. Nursing Ethics 1, 86-95.

Edney, J. (1974) Human territoriality. Psychological Bulletin 81 (12), 959-975.

Eduskunnan oikeusasiamiehen kertomus (1973) Helsinki: Valtion painatuskeskus.

Edwards, S. (1998) An anthropological interpretation of nurses' and patients' perceptions of the use of space and touch. Journal of Advanced Nursing 28, 809-817.

Edwards, S.J.L., Lilford, R.J., Thornton, J. & Hewison, J. (1998) Informed consent for clinical trials: in search of the "best" method. Social Science and Medicine 47 (11), 1825-1840.

Ekman S-L. & Nordberg A. (1988) The autonomy of demented patients: interviews with caregivers. Journal of Medical Ethics 14, 184-187.

Elander, G., Drechsler, K & Persson, K.W. (1993) Ethical dilemmas in long-term care settings: interviews with nurses in Sweden and England. International Journal of Nursing Studies 30 (1), 91-97.

Elander, G. & Hermerén, G. (1989) Autonomy and paternalistic behaviour in care. Scandinavian Journal of Caring Sciences 3 (4), 153-159.

Eleftheroudakis (1965) Encyclopedia dictionary. Eleftheroudakis, 11, 888, Athens.

Eliasson, A. & Poropatich, R. (1998) Performance improvement in telemedicine: the essential elements. Military Medicine 163 (8), 530-535.

Elliott, J. (1982) Living in Hospital. London: King Edward's Hospital Fund for London.

Emanuel, E.J. (1987) A communal vision of care for incompetent patients. Hastings Center Report October/November, 15-20.

Emerson, J. (1973) Behavior in private places: sustaining definitions of reality in gynecological examination. In R. Wertz (ed.) Readings on ethical and social issues in biomedicine. Englewood Cliffs: Prentice Hall, 221-231.

Ende, J., Kazis, L., Ash, A. & Moskowitz, M.A. (1989) Measuring patients' desire for autonomy: decision-making and information seeking preferences among medical patients. Journal of General Internal Medicine 4 (1), 23-30.

Ende, J., Kazis, L. & Moskowitz, M.A. (1990) Preference for autonomy when patients are physicians. Journal of General Internal Medicine 5 (6), 506-509.

Etzioni, A. (1998) HIV testing of infants: privacy and public health. Health Affairs Millwood 17 (4), 170-183.

European Community Directive 91/507/EEC. London: HMSO.

Faden, R., & Beauchamp, T. (1986) A history and theory of informed consent. New York: Oxford University Press.

Faletti, M. (1984) Human factors research and functional environments for aged. In I. Altman, M. Lawton & J. Wohlwill (eds.) Elderly people and the environment. Human Behavior and Environment, Advances in Theory and Research Volume 7. New York: Plenum Press, 191-237.

Falk, S. & Woods, N. (1973) Hospital noise – levels and potential health hazards. New England Journal of Medicine 289 (15), 774-781.

Farrell, G.A. (1991) How accurately do nurses perceive patients' needs? A comparison of general and psychiatric settings. Journal of Advanced Nursing 16, 1062-1070.

The Finnish Ministry of Social Affairs and Health (1996) Three years in force: has the Finnish act on the status and rights of patients materialized? Helsinki: Publication of the Ministry 4.

Fitten, L. & Waite, M. (1990) Impact of medical hospitalization on treatment decision-making capacity in the elderly. Archives of Internal Medicine 150 (8), 1717-1721.

Frantzeskaki, I. (1990) The penitentiary system. Athens.

Friedlander, W. (1982) The basis of privacy and autonomy in medical practice. A model. Social Science and Medicine 16 (19), 1709-1718.

Friend, B. (1996) Risky business? Nursing Times 92 (30), 26-27.

Frith, L. (Ed.) (1998a) Ethics and midwifery. Issues in contemporary practice. Oxford: Butterworth-Heineman.

Frith, L. (1998b) Reproductive technologies and midwifery. In Ethics and Midwifery. L. Frith (ed.) Issues in contemporary practice. Oxford: Butterworth-Heineman, 170-188.

Fromer, M.J. (1981) Ethical issues in health care. St. Louis: CV Mosby.

Fry, S.T. (1989) Ethical issues in clinical research. Informed consent and risks versus benefits in the treatment of primary hypertension. Nursing Clinics of North America 24 (4), 1033-1039.

Fry, S.T. (1995) Ethik in der Pflegepraxis. Anleitung für die ethische Entscheidungsfindung. Eschborn:

DBfK-Verlag.

Fulbrook, P. (1994) Assessing the mental competence of patients and relatives. Journal of Advanced Nursing 20, 457-461.

Funk, W. (1950) Word origins and their romantic stories. New York: Grosset & Dunlap.

Gadow, S. (1989a) An ethical case for self-determination. Seminars in Oncology Nursing, 5 (2), 99-101.

Gadow S. (1989b) Clinical subjectivity. Advocacy with silent patients. Nursing Clinics of North America 24, 535-541.

Gafo, J. (1994) Etica y Legislación en Enfermeria. Madrid: Editorial Universitas.

Gainsborough, H. (1970) Privacy and patient care. British Hospital Journal and Social Service Review 24, 751-752.

Gale, B.J. (1989) Advocacy for elderly autonomy: a challenge for community health nurses. Journal of Community Health Nursing 6 (4), 191-197.

Gambone, J.C. & Reiter, R.C. (1997) Hysterectomy: improving the patient's decision-making process. Clinical Obstetrics and Gynecology 40 (4), 868-877.

Gardner, R. & Lundsgaarde, H. (1994) Evaluating of user acceptance of a clinical expert systems. Journal of the American Medical Informatics Association 1 (6), 428-438.

George, J. & Quattrone, M. (1985) Search for patient identification: an invasion of privacy. Journal of Emergency Nursing 11 (6), 335-336.

Geden, E. & Begeman, A. (1981) Personal space preferences of hospitalized adults. Research in Nursing and Health 4 (2), 237-241.

Generalitat de Catalunya (1997) Guía de Recomanacions sobre el consentiment informat. Departament de Sanitat i Seguretat Social. Barcelona.

Gifford, R. (1987) Environmental psychology, principles and practice. Boston: Allyn and Bacon.

Gillett, G.R. (1989) Informed consent and moral integrity. Journal of Medical Ethics 15 (3), 117- 123.

Gillon, R. (1986) Autonomy and the principle of respect for autonomy. British Medical Journal 290, 1806 - 1808.

Gioiella, E. (1978) The relationships between slowness of response, state anxiety, social isolation and self-esteem, and preferred personal space in the elderly. Journal of Gerontological Nursing 4 (1), 40-43.

Gracia, D. (1989) Fundamentos de Bioética. Madrid: Eudema.

Gracia, D. (1993) The intellectual basis of Bioethics in Southern European countries. Bioethics 7 (2/3), 97-107.

Grafter, H. & Rowan, C. (1998) Ethical issues in maternity care. In W. Tadd (ed.) Ethical issues in nursing and midwifery practice. Perspectives from Europe. London: MacMillan, 103-123.

Graw, M. (1995) Das Selbstbestimmungsrecht des Patienten. Aus dem Institut für gerichtliche Medizin der Universität Tübingen. Medizinische Welt 46 (3), 165-171.

Griffiths, P. (1995) Progress in measuring nursing outcomes. Journal of Advanced Nursing 21, 1092-1100.

Gross, H. (1971) Privacy and autonomy. In J. Pennock & J. Chapman (eds.) Privacy. New York: Atherton Press, 169-181.

Grossman, S.A., Piantadosi, S. & Covahey, C. (1994) Are informed consent forms that describe clinical oncology research protocols readable by most patients and their families? Journal of Clinical Oncology 12 (10), 2211 - 2215.

Grundner, T. (1980) On the readability of surgical consent form. New England Journal of Medicine 302, 900-902.

Gryparis, I. (1997) Plato Politeia. Zacharopoulos Vol A. Athens.

Guttman-McGabe, C. (1997) Telemedicine's imperilled future? Funding, reimbursement, licensing and privacy hurdles face a development of technology. Journal of Contemporary Health Law Policy 14, 161-186.

van den Haag, E. (1971) On privacy. In J. Pennock & J. Chapman (eds.) Privacy. New York: Atherton Press, 149-168.

Hall, E. (1959) The hidden dimension. New York: Anchor books.

Hall, E. (1966) The hidden dimension. New York: Doubleday and Company.

Hall, E. (1970) The anthropoloogy of space: An organizing model. In H. Prohansky, W. Ittleson & L. Rivlin (eds.) Environmental psychology. Man and his physical setting. New York: Hotel, Rinehart and Winston.

Hall J. & Dornan M. (1988) What patients like about their medical care and how often they are asked: A meta-analysis of the satisfaction literature. Social Science and Medicine 27, 935-939.

Hallborg, R. (1986) Principles of liberty and the right to privacy. Law and Philosophy 5, 175-218.

Hamaguchi, K. (1998) Role of nursing informed consent. Hokkaido Journal of medical Science 73 (1), 21-25. [In Japanise, English abstract]

Hammerschmidt, D. & Keane, M. (1992) Institutional Review Board (IRB) review lacks impact on the readability of consent forms for research. The American Journal of the Medical Sciences 304 (6), 348-351.

Hannikainen, L. (toim.) (1992) Eettiset säännöt. Åbo Akademin ihmisoikeusinstituutti. Turku: Åbo Akademis tryckeri.

Hart, G. (1980) Maternal attitudes in prepared and unprepared cesarean deliveries. JOGN Nursing 9 (49), 243-245.

Haslam, P. (1970) Noise in hospitals: its effect on the patient. Nursing Clinics of North America 5, 715-724.

Hayter, J. (1981) Territoriality as a universal need. Journal of Advanced Nursing 6, 79-85.

HE (1986) Hallituksen esitys henkilörekisterilaiksi No 49/1986. 1.10.1986. Hallituksen esitys, Asiakirjat A1.

HE (1991) Hallituksen esitys eduskunnalle laiksi potilaan asemasta ja oikeuksista No 185/1991. Asiakirjat A4.

Headings, V.E. (1997) Revisiting foundations of autonomy and beneficence in genetic counseling. Genetic Counselling 8 (4), 291-294.

Health Plan of Catalonia 1996-98 (1998) (Pla de Salut de Catalunya 1996-98) The Ministry of Health of Catalonia. Barcelona, Spain.

Heater B., Becker A. & Olson R. (1988) Nursing interventions and patient outcomes: a meta-analysis of studies. Nursing Research 37, 303-307.

Helmchen, H. (1997) Einwilligung nach Aufklärung ("informed consent") in der Psychiatrie – Europäische Standards und Unterschiede, Probleme und Empfehlungen. Originalarbeit Biomed 1 Projekt, Vortrag von 1995 in Berlin. Fortschritte der Neurologie/Psychiatrie 65 (1), 23-33.

Henderson, V. (1969) Basic principles of nursing care. Geneva: International Council of Nurses.

Hendricks, A. (1997) Genetics, human rights and employment from American and European perspectives. Medical Law 16 (3), 557-565.

Herbert, V. (1980) Informed consent - a legal evaluation. Cancer 46, 1042-1044.

Hertz, J.E. (1996) Conceptualization of perceived enactment of autonomy in the elderly. Issues in Mental Health Nursing 17, 261-273.

Hertz, D.A., Looman, J.E. & Lewis, S.K. (1992) Informed consent: is it a myth? Neurosurgery 30 (3), 453-458.

Hewison, A. (1995) Nurses' power in interactions with patients. Journal of Advanced Nursing 21, 75-82.

Higgs, P., MacDonald, L. & Ward, M. (1992) Responses to the institution among elderly patients in hospital long-stay care. Social Science and Medicine 35 (3), 287-293.

Hiller, J. (1981) Compuers, medical records, and the right to privacy. Journal of Health Polit Policy Law 6 (3), 463-487.

Hilton, B. (1976) Quantity and quality of patients' sleep and sleep-disturbing factors in a respiratory intensive care unit. Journal of Advanced Nursing 1, 453-468.

Hines, P. (1985) "One's own place": a case study on territorial behavior. Nursing Forum XXII (1), 31-33.

Hofmann, I. (1996) Aufgaben einer Pflegeethik - als Beispiel - Wahrhaftigkeit im Umgang mit kranken/sterbenden Menschen. Medizinische Schriften. Heft 9. Dortmund: Humanitas Verlag.

Hoge, S. (1995) Proposed federal legistlation jeopardizes patient privacy. Bulletin of the American Academy of Psychiatry and Law 23 (4), 495-500.

Hopper, K.D., Houts, P.S., McCauslin, M.A., Matthews, Y.L. & Sefczek, R.J. (1992) Patients' attitudes toward informed consent for intravenous contrast media. Investigative Radiology 27, 362-366.

Hopper, K.D., Zajdel, M., Hulse, S.F., Yoanidis, N.R., TenHave, T.R., Labuski, M.R., Houts, P.S., Bresinger, C.M. & Hartman, D.S. (1994) Interactive method of informing patients of the risks of intravenous contrast media. Radiology 192, 67-71.

Hord, C. & Delano, G. (1994) The midwife's role in abortion care. Midwifery 10 (3), 131-141.

Horner, J. (1998) Research, ethics and privacy: the limits of knowledge. Public Health 112 (4), 217-220.

Horowitz, A., Silverstone, B.M. & Reinhardt, J.P. (1991) A conceptual and empirical exploration of personal autonomy issues within family caregiving relationships. Gerontologist 31 (1), 23-31.

Houghton, D., Williams, S., Bennett, J., Back, G. & Jones, A. (1997) Informed consent: patients' and junior doctors' perceptions of the consent procedure. Clinical Otolaryngology 22 (6), 515-518.

Hovi, S-L. (1990) Fyysinen ympäristö potilaan toiminnan rajoittajana. Tutkielma, Turun yliopisto. Turku: Hoitotieteen laitos.

Howard, O.M., Fairclough, D.L., Daniels, E.R. & Emanuel, E.J. (1997) Physician desire for euthanasia and assisted suicide: would physicians practice what they preach? Journal of Clinical Oncology 15 (2), 428-432.

Hutson McDaniel, M. & Blaha, J.D. (1991) Patients' recall of preoperative instruction for informed consent for an operation. The Journal of Bone and Joint Surgery 73A (2), 160-162.

Illhardt, F.J. (1985) Medizinische Ethik. Ein Arbeitsbuch Medizinische Ethik. Berlin: Springer Verlag.

Ilveskivi, P. (1997a) Potilaan oikeusasema tiedonsaantioikeuden näkökulmasta. Kansaneläkelaitos. Sosiaali- ja terveysturvan tutkimuksia. Helsinki: Hakapaino Oy.

Ilveskivi, P. (1997b) Potilaan tiedonsaantioikeus. Teoksessa Lääkintäoikeudellisia kirjoituksia. Eripainos Lakimies-aikakauskirjan lääkintäoikeuden teemanumerosta 6/1997. Lääkintäoikeuden julkaisuja 1, Helsingin yliopisto, Rikos- ja prosessioikeuden sekä oikeuden yleistieteiden laitos, Helsinki, 774-805.

Ingham, R. (1978) Privacy and psychology. In J. Young (ed.) Privacy. John Wiley & Sons, Chichester, 35-57.

Inglis, S. & Farnill, D. (1993) The effects of providing preoperative statistical anaesthetic-risk information. Anaesthesia and Intensive Care 21 (6), 799-805.

Insel, P. (1978) Too close for comfort. Englewood Cliffs: Prentice-Hall.

Intimate examinations (1997) Report of a Working Party. London: RCOG Press.

Ip, M., Gilligan T., Koenig, B. & Raffin, T.A. (1998) Ethical decision-making in critical care in Hong Kong. Critical Care Medicine 26 (3), 447-451.

Iseminger, K.A. & Lewis, M.A. (1998) Ethical challenges in treating mother and fetus when cancer complicates pregnancy. Obstetrics and Gynecology Clinics of North America 25 (2), 273-285.

Isola, A. & Laitinen, P. (1995) Hoitotyön sisältö ja hoitohenkilöstön työajankäyttö geriatrisella osastolla. Hoitotiede 7 (5), 249-255.

Jablonski, D., Mosley, M., Byrd, J., Schwallie, D. & Nattinger, A. (1991) Informed consent for patient transfers to a Veterans affairs medical center. Journal of General Internal Medicine 6 (3), 229-232.

Jang, G. (1992) Autonomy of institutionalized elderly. Residents' and staff perception. Canadian Journal of Aging 11 (3), 249-261.

Jantunen, K. Puumalainen, A., Suominen, T. & Leino-Kilpi, H. (1994) Onko sairaalassa yksityisyyttä? Turun yliopisto, Hoitotieteen laitos, Julkaisuja A 5. Turku: Turun yliopisto.

Jecker, N.1991 (Ed.) Aging and ethics. New Jersey: Human Press, Clifton.

Jensen, A.B. (1990) Informed consent. Historical background and present-day problems. Ugeskr Laeger 152, 3591-3593.

Jensen, A., Madsen, B., Andersen, P. & Rose, C. (1993) Information for cancer patients entering a clinical trial - an evaluation of an information strategy. European Journal of Cancer 29A (16), 2235-2238.

Jezewski, M., Scherer, Y., Miller, C. & Battista, E. (1993) Consenting to DNR: critical care nurses' interactions with patients and family members. American Journal of Critical Care 2 (4), 302-309.

Johnson, F. (1978) Territorial behavior of nursing home residents. Issues in Mental Health Nursing 1 (Spring 1978), 44-52.

Johnson, F. (1979) Response to territorial intrusion by nursing home residents. Advances in Nursing Science 1 (4), 21-34.

Johnston, J. (1988) Preserving privacy and confidentiality for the emergency patient. Emergency Nursing Reports 3 (4), 1-8.

Johnstone, M-J. (1989) Bioethics: a nursing perspective. Sydney: Saunders.

Johnstone, M.J. (1998) In J. Richardson & I. Webber (Hrsg.) Ethische Aspekte der Kinderkrankenpflege. Wiesbaden: Ullstein Medical, 3-4.

Jubelirer, S., Linton, J. & Magnetti, S. (1994) Reading versus comprehension: implications for patient education and consent in an outpatient oncology clinic. Journal of Cancer Education 9, 26-29.

Juchli, L. (1994) Pflege: Praxis und Theorie der Gesundheits- und Krankenpflege. 7. neubearbeitete Auflage. Stuttgart: G. Thieme Verlag.

Justin, R. (1989) Cost containment forces physicians into ethical and quality of care compromises. Theoretical Medicine 10 (3), 231-238.

Kalkas, H. & Sarvimäki, A. (1994) Hoitotyön etiikan perusteet. SHKS. Keuruu: Otava.

Kanerva, A-M., Suominen, T. & Leino-Kilpi, H. (1999) Informed consent in short-stay surgery. Nursing Ethics 6 (6), 483-493.

Kant, I. (1997) Kritique of practical reason. Mary Gregory, M. (ed.) Cambridge: Cambridge University Press.

Katz, V.L., Seeds, J.W., Albright, S.G., Lingley, L.H. & Lincoln-Boyea, B. (1991) Role of ultrasound and informed consent in the evaluation of elevated maternal serum alpha-fetoprotein. American Journal of Perinatology 8 (2), 73-76.

Katzko, M.W., Steverink, N., Dittmann, K.F. & Herrera, R.R. (1998) The self-concept of the elderly: a cross-cultural comparison. Internal Journal of Aging and Human Development 46 (3), 171-187.

Kaufert, J. & O'Neil, J. (1990) Biomedical rituals and informed consent: native Canadians and the negotiation of clinical trust. In G. Weisz (ed.) Social science perspectives on medical ethics. Philadelphia: University of Pennsylvania Press, 41-64.

Kaufman, C.L. (1983) Informed consent and patient decision making: two decades of research. Social Sciences Medicine 17, 1657 - 1664.

Kayser-Jones, J. (1990) The use of nasogastric feeding tubes in nursing homes: patient, family and health care provider perspectives. The Gerontologist 30, 469-479.

Keefe, M. (1984) The effect of the hospital environment on newborn state behavior and maternal sleep.Dissertation Abstracts International 45, 1429 B. University Microfilms No 8418015.

Keenan, J. (1999) A concept analysis of autonomy. Journal of Advanced Nursing 29 (3), 556-562.

Kellermann, A. & Ackerman, T. (1988) Interhospital patient transfer: the case for informed consent. New England Journal of Medicine 319, 643-646.

Kelly, W., Krause, E., Krowinski, W., Small, T. & Drane, J. (1990) National survey of ethical issues presented to drug information centers. American Journal of Hospital Pharmagology 47 (10), 2245-2250.

Kelvin, P. (1973) A social psychological examination of privacy. British Journal of Social and Clinical Psychology 12, 248-261.

Kennedy, I. (1992) Consent to treatment. In C. Dyer (ed.) Doctors, patients and the law. Oxford: Blackwell Science Ltd, 44-71.

Kennett, A. (1986) Informed consent: a patient's view. Professional Nurse 2 (3), 75-77.

Kerr, J. (1982) An overview of theory and research related to space use in hospitals. Western Journal of Nursing Research 4 (4), 395-405.

Kerr, J. (1985) Space use, privacy, and territoriality. Western Journal of Nursing Research 7 (2), 199-219.

Kerrigan, D.D., Thevasagayam, R.S., Woods, T.O., McWelch, I., Thomas, W.E.G., Shorthouse, A.J., & Dennison, A.R. (1993) Who's afraid of informed consent? British Medical Journal 506, 298-300.

Kim, H.N., Gates, E. & Lo, B. (1998) What hysterectomy: patients what to know about the roles of residents and medical students in their care. Academic Medicine 73 (3), 339-341.

Koergaonkar, G. (1992) Consent to treatment: what value consent forms? British Journal of Hospital Medicine 47 (11), 836-837.

Kokkonen, P. (1993) Informed consent: a Nordic perspective. Medicine and Law 12, 583-592.

Kokkonen P. (1994) The new Finnish law on the Status and Rights of a Patient. European Journal of Health Law 1, 127-135.

Kollwitz, A. A. (1997) Entwicklung der Patientenautonomie – Herausforderung für den Ärztestand. In: Körner, U. & Neumann, G. (Hrsg.) Patientautonomie und Humanes Sterben. Kongressbericht. Medizinische Schriften. Heft 14/15. Dortmund: Humanitas Verlag, 15-25.

Komiteanmietintö (1982) Komiteanmietintö No 65, 1982. Terveydenhuollon oikeussuojatoimikunnan mietintö II: ehdotus laiksi potilaan oikeuksista 1982:65. Helsinki: Valtion painatuskeskus.

Korhonen, R. (1994) Eutanasia - hyvä kuolema ja kuolemisen vaikeus. Lapin yliopiston oikeustieteellisiä julkaisuja C 18 (Euthanasia - good death and the difficulty of dying). Rovaniemi: Pandeca Oy.

Koutselinis, A. & Michalodimitrakis, M. (1984) Medical responsibility. Athens: Gutenberg.

Kranich, C. (1997) Patientenrechte und Patientenunterstützung in Europa. Baden Baden: Nomos Verlag.

Kruse, J. (1984) Long-term reactions of women to electronic fetal monitoring during labor. Journal of Family Practice 18 (4), 543-548.

Krynski, M., Tymchuk, A. & Ouslander, J. (1994) How informed can consent be? New light on comprehension among elderly people making decisions about enteral tube feeding. The Gerontologist 34 (1), 36-43.

Kuuppelomäki, M. & Lauri, S. (1989) Eettiset ongelmat iäkkäiden terminaalivaiheessa olevien potilaiden syöttämisessä. Hoitotiede 1 (2), 56-60.

Körner, U. (1994) Autonomie und Menschenwürde in der Medizin – ethische und rechtliche Fragen. Zeitschrift für Ärztliche Fortbildung 88, 731-732.

Lahti, R. (1994) Towards a comprehensive legislation governing the rights of patients: the Finnish experience. In L. Westerhäll & C. Phillips (eds.) Patient's Rights. Informed consent, access and equality. Göteborg: Graphic Systems, 207-221.

Lahti, R. (1995) The Finnish Patient Injury Compensation System. In S.A.M. McLean, Law reform and Medical injury litigation. Dartmouth. Cambridge: The University Press, 147-162.

Lahti, R. (1997) Lääkintäoikeus: kehittyvä uusi tieteenala. Teoksessa Lääkintäoikeudellisia kirjoituksia. Erillispainos Lakimies-aikakauskirjan lääkintäoikeuden teemanumerosta 6/1997, 753-759.

Lalli, A. (1980) Contrast media reactions: data analysis and hypothesis. Radiology 134, 1-12.

Lalli, A. & Greenstreet, R. (1981) Reactions to contrast media: testing the CNS hypothesis. Radiology 138, 47-49.

Lambe, H., Hopper, K. & Matthews, Y. (1992) Use of informed consent for ionic and nonionic contrast media. Radiology 184, 145-148.

Lane, P. (1989) Nurse-client perceptions: the doubled standard of touch. Issues in Mental Health Nursing 10, 1-13.

Lane, P. (1990) A measure of clients' perceptions about intrusions of territory and personal space by nurses. In O. Strickland & C. Waltz (eds.) Measurement of nursing outcomes. Vol 4, Measuring client self-care and coping skills. New York: Springer, 199-218.

Lang, L. & Nikkonen, M. (1994) Kätilöiden hoitokulttuuri ja synnyttäjien hoitoa koskevia odotuksia ja kokemuksia. Hoitotiede 6 (3), 107-115.

Laufer, R. & Wolfe, M. (1977) Privacy as a concept and a social issue: a multidimensional development theory. Journal of Social Issues 33 (3), 22-42.

Lavelle-Jones, C., Byrne, D.J., Rice, P. & Cushieri, A. (1993) Factors affecting quality of informed consent. British Medical Journal 306 (3), 885-890.

Leenen, H. (1994) The rights of patients in Europe. European Journal of Health Law 1, 5-13.

Van der Leer, O.F.C. (1994) The use of personal data for medical research: how to deal with new European privacy standards. International Journal of Bio-Medical Computing 35 (suppl 1), 87-95.

Leibman, M. (1970) The effects of sex and race norms on personal space. Environment and behavior 2 (2), 208-246.

Leighton, B., Bauman, J., Seltzer, J. & Menduke, H. (1987) The effect of a detailed anesthesia consent form on patient recall and anxiety (Abstract). Anesthesiology 67, A567.

Leino-Kilpi, H. (1990) Good nursing care. On what basis? Acta Universitatis Turkuensis, Series Medica-Odontologica, D 49. University of Turku. Turku: Kirjapaino Pika Oy.

Leino-Kilpi, H., Iire, L., Suominen, T., Vuorenheimo, J. & Välimäki M. (1993) Client and information: a literature review. Journal of Clinical Nursing 2, 331-340.

Leino-Kilpi, H. & Kurittu, K. (1995) Patients' rights in hospital. An empirical investigation in Finland. Nursing Ethics 2 (2), 103-113.

Leino-Kilpi, H., Nyrhinen, T. & Katajisto, J. (1997) Patients' rights in laboratory examinations: do they realize? Nursing Ethics 4 (6), 451-464.

Leino-Kilpi, H. & Vuorenheimo, J. (1992) Patient satisfaction as an indicator of the quality of nursing care. Vård i Norden 12, 22-28.

Leist, A. (1994) Patientenautonomie und ärztliche Verantwortung. Zeitschrift für Ärztliche Fortbildung 88, 733-742.

Levy-Leboyer, C. (1982) Psychology and environment. Beverly Hills: Sage Publications.

Lewis, K. (1995) How to foster self-determination. Practical ways nursing home staff can empower their residents. Health Progress November-December, 42-44.

Ley, P. (1982) Giving information to patients. In J.R. Eiser (ed.) Social psychology and behavioural medicine. New York: Wiley, 339-373.

Liljeström, M. (1993) Potilaan oikeudet ihmisoikeuksina ja perusoikeuksina. Sosiaalinen Aikakauskirja 2, 10-14.

Lind, S., DelVecchio, G. & Seidel, S. (1989) Telling the diagnosis of cancer. Journal of Clinical Oncology 75, 5583-598.

Lindley, R. (1991) Informed consent and the ghost of Bolam. In M. Brazier & M. Lobjoit (eds.) Protecting the vulnerable. Autonomy and consent in health care. London: Routledge, 134-149.

Lindqvist, M. (1980) Potilaan suostumuksen periaate ja sen rajat. Suomen Lääkärilehti 35, 1552-1557.

Little, K. (1965) Personal space. Journal of Experimental Social Psychology 1, 237-247.

Liukkonen, A. (1990) Dementoituneen potilaan perushoito laitoksessa. Turun yliopiston julkaisuja C 81. Turun yliopisto. Turku: Kirjapaino Pika Oy.

Lofmark, R. & Nilstun, T. (1998) Informing patients and relatives about do-not-resuscitate decisions. Attitudes of cardiologists and nurses in Sweden. Journal of Internal Medicine 243 (3), 191-195.

Lonsdale, M. & Hutchinson, G. (1991) Patients' desire for information about anaesthesia. Scottish and Canadian attitudes. Anaesthesia 46, 410-412.

Louis, M. (1981) Personal space boundary needs of elderly persons: an empirical study. Journal of Gerontological Nursing 7 (7), 395-400.

Lydon-Rochelle, M. & Albers, L. (1993) Research trends in the Journal of Nurse-Midwifery 1987-1992. Journal of Nurse-Midwifery 38 (6), 343-348.

Lyman, S. & Scott, M. (1967) Territoriality: a neglected sociological dimension. Journal of Social Problems 15 (2), 236-249.

Lynöe, N., Sandlund, M., Dahlqvist, G. & Jacobsson, L. (1991) Informed consent: study of quality of information given to participants in a clinical trial. British Journal of Medicine 303 (14), 610-613.

Lääkärin etiikka (1992). Suomen Lääkäriliitto. Forssa: Forssan kirjapaino Oy.

Lääkärin etiikka (1996) Suomen Lääkäriliitto. Forssa: Forssan kirjapaino Oy.

Lötjönen, S. (1998) The protection of human subjects in medical research in Finland. In T. Modeen (ed.) Finnish National Reports. To the XVTH Congress of the International Academy of Comparative Law. Helsinki: Finnish Lawyers' Publishing, Kauppakaari Oy, Multiprint, 51-72.

MacCormick, D. (1974) Privacy: a problem of definition. British Journal of Law and Society 1 (1), 75-78.

MacDaniel, C. & Nash, J. (1990) Compendium of instruments measuring patient satisfaction with nursing care. Quality Review Bulletin 16, 181-188.

MacIntyre, A. (1977) Patients as agents. In S.F. Spicker & H.T. Engelhardt (eds.) Philosophical medical ethics: its nature and significance. Dordrecht: D. Reidel Publishing Company, 197-212.

Magaziner, J. (1988) Living density and psychopathology: a re-examination of the negative model. Psychological Medicine 18 (2), 419-431.

Malin, N., & Teasdale, K. (1991) Caring versus empowerment: considerations for nursing practice. Journal of Advanced Nursing 16, 657 - 662.

Mallon-Palmer, M. (1980) Personal space theories: lessons for nurses. The Australian Nurses Journal 10 (5), 36-38.

Mander, R. (1998) Failure to deliver: ethical issues relating to epidural analgesia in uncomplicated labour. In L. Frith (ed.) Ethics and midwifery: issues in contemporary practice. Great Britain: Butterworth Heinemann, 51-71.

Mandilaras, V. (1994) Hippocrates varia: general medicine. Athens: Kaktos.

Manessis, A. & Papadimitriou, G. (1986) The Greek Constitution of 1975/1986. Athens: Sakkoula.

Marchette, L., Box, N., Hennessy, M., Wasserlau, M., Arnall, B., Copeland, D & Habib, K. (1993) Nurses' perceptions of the support of patient autonomy in do-not-resuscitate (DNR) decisions. International Journal of Nursing Studies 30 (1), 37-49

Mark, J.S. & Spiro, H. (1990) Informed consent for colonscopy. A prospective study. Archives of Internal Medicine 150 (4), 777-780.

Marieb, E.N. (1992) Human anatomy and physiology. (2nd ed.). California: Benjamin/Cummings.

Markova, I. (1995) Human agency and the quality of life: a theoretical overview. In I. Markova & R. Farr (eds.) Representations of health, illness and handicap. Amsterdam: Harwood Academic Publishers, 191-204.

Markus, K. (1996a) Eigener Wunsch oder wider Willen, Teil 1. Das Selbstbestimmungsrecht bei alten Menschen. Altenpflege 5, 363-365.

Markus, K. (1996b) Eigener Wunsch oder wider Willen, Teil 2. Selbstbestimmung bei der Verwendung und Verwaltung des Barbetrages zur persönlichen Verfügung. Altenpflege 5, 363-365.

Marr, H. & Pirie, M. (1990) Protecting privacy. Nursing Times 86, 58-59.

Marshall, N. (1974) Dimensions of privacy preferences. Multivariate Behavioral Research 19 (3), 255-271.

Martens, E. (1995) Ethik-Kodex, Ethische Grundregeln der Altenpflege. Gransee: Fachseminar Altenpflege.

Massué, J-P. (1998) Preface. In Concil of Europe. The human rights, ethical and moral dimensions of health care. 120 practical case studies. European Network of Scientific Co-operation on Medicine and Human Rights. Councul of Europe Publishing. Germany, 11-17.

Mason, J.K. & McCall Smith, R.A. (1994) Law and medical Ethics. (4th ed.). Edinburgh: Butterworths.

Mattiasson, A-C. & Andersson, L. (1994) Staff attitude and experience in dealing with rational nursing home patients who refuse to eat and drink. Journal of Advanced Nursing 20 (5), 822-827.

Mattiasson, A-C. & Andersson, L. (1995a) Nursing homes staff attitudes to ethical conflicts with respect to patient autonomy and paternalism. Nursing Ethics 2 (2), 115-130.

Mattiasson, A.C., & Andersson, L. (1995b) Organisational environment and the support of patient autonomy in nursing home care. Journal of Advanced Nursing 22, 1149-1157.

Mattiasson, A-C. & Hemberg, M. (1998) Intimacy - meeting needs and respecting privacy in the care of elderly people: what is a good moral attitude on the part of the nurse/carer? Nursing Ethics 5, 527-534.

May, C. (1995) Patient autonomy and the politics of professional relationships. Journal of Advanced Nursing 21 (1), 83-87.

Mazaux, J.M., Masson, F., Levin, H.S., Alaoui, P., Maurette, P. & Barat, M. (1997) Long-term neuropsychological outcome and loss of social autonomy after traumatic brain injury. Archives of Physical Medicine and Rehabilitation 78 (12), 1316-1320.

McCloskey, H. (1971) The political ideal of privacy. Philosophical Quarterly 21, 305-306.

McCormack, B. (1993) How to promote quality of care and preserve patient autonomy. British Journal of Nursing 2 (6), 338-341.

McCracken, A. (1987) Emotional impact of possession loss. Journal of Gerontological Nursing 13 (2), 14-19.

McElmurry, B.J. & Zabrocki, E. (1989) Ethical concerns in caring for older women in the community. Nursing Clinics of North America 24 (4), 1041-1050.

McWilliam, C., Belle Brown, J., Carmichael, J. & Lehman, J. (1994) A new perspective on threatened autonomy in elderly persons: the disempowering process. Social Science and Medicine 38 (2), 327-338.

Meisel, A. & Roth, L.H. (1981) What we do and do not know about informed consent. The Journal of the

American Medical Association 246 (21), 2473-2477.

Meisenheimer, J. (1982) Boundaries of personal space. Image XIV (1), 16-19.

Meisenheimer, C. (Ed.) (1992) Improving quality. A guide to effective programs. Gaithersburg, MD: Aspen.

Mello, M. & Jenkinson, C. (1998) Comparison of medical and nursing students' attitudes to resuscitation and patient autonomy between a British and an Americal teaching hospitals. Social Science and Medicine 46 (3), 415-424.

Meredith, B. (1987) Maybe I'm old but I'm still a person. Health Service Journal, May, 1318-1319.

Merkouris, A., Ifantopoulos, J., Lanara, V. & Lemonidou, C. (1999a) Patient satisfaction: a key concept for evaluating and improving nursing services. Journal of Nursing Management 7, 19-29.

Merkouris, A., Ifantopoulos, J., Lanara, V. & Lemonidou, C. (1999b) Patient satisfaction: instrumentation. Journal of Nursing Management 7, 91-100.

Meyers grosses Taschenlexikon (1992) Band 20. Mannheim: Bibliographisches Institut & F.A. Brockhaus AG.

Michielutte, R., Bahnson, J. & Beal, P. (1990) Readability of the public education literature on cancer prevention and detection. Journal of Cancer Education 5, 55-61.

Milholland, D. (1994) Privacy and confidentiality of patient information. Challenges for nursing. Journal of Nursing Administration 24 (2), 19-24.

Miller, J. (1992) Analysis of coping with illness. In J. Miller (ed.) Coping with chronic illness. Philadelphia: F.A. Davis, 19-49.

Minckley, B. (1968) Space and place in patient care. American Journal of Nursing 68 (3), 510-516.

Moehr, J. (1998) Informatics in the service of health, a look to the future. Methods of Information in Medicine 37 (2), 165-170.

Moos, R. & Lemke, S. (1984) Supportive residential settings for older people. In I. Altman, M. Lawton & J. Wohlwill (eds.) Elderly people and the environment. Human Behavior and Environment, Advances in Theory and Research, Volume 7. New York: Plenum Press, 159-190.

Morrow, G. (1980) How readable are subject informed consent forms? Journal of American Medical Association 244, 56-58.

Morse, J.M. (1991) Negotiating commitment and involvement in the nurse-patient relationship. Journal of Advanced Nursing 16, 455-468.

Muller, J. & Desmond, B. (1992) Ethical dilemmas in a cross-cultural context: a Chinese example. Western Journal of Medicine 157, 323-327.

Muss, H., White, D., Michielutte, R., Richards, F., Cooper, M., Williams, S., Stuart, J. & Spurr, C. (1979) Written information consent in patients with breast cancer. Cancer 43 (4), 1549-1556.

Muyskens, J. (1982) Moral problems in nursing: a philosophical investigation. Totowa: Rowman and Littlefield.

Nelson, M. & Paluck, R. (1980) Territorial markings, self-concept, and mental status of the institutionalized elderly. The Gerontologist 20 (1), 96-98.

Neptune, S.M., Hopper, K.D. & Matthews, Y.L. (1994) Risks associated with the use of IV contrast material: analysis of patients' awareness. American Journal of Roentgenology 162 (2), 451-454.

Newman, D.L. & Brown, R.D. (1996) Applied ethics for program evaluation. Thousand Oaks: Sage Publications.

Newton, J., Hawes, R., Jamidar, P. Harig, J. & Lehman, G. (1994) Survey of informed consent for endoscopic retrograde cholangiopancreatography. Digestive Diseases and Sciences 39 (8), 1714-1718.

Nicholas, D. (1988) Socially valid problem situations in outpatient cancer therapy. Journal of Psychosocial Oncology 6 (1/2) 21-29.

Niedz, B.A. (1998) Correlates of hospitalized patients' perceptions of service quality. Research in Nursing and Health 21 (4), 339-349.

Niemi, A. (1994) Riisuttuna - potilaiden kokemat eheyden uhat ja selviytyminen urologisten tautien ja naistentautien osastolla. Pro gradu-tutkielma. Tampere: Tampereen yliopisto.

Nightingale, F. (1980) Notes on nursing. Edinburgh: Churchill Livingstone. (Originally published by Harrison and Sons in 1859).

Nikkilä, J. (1998) Terveydenhuollon kehittämisprojekti. Selvitysmiesraportti 1, terveydenhuollon toimivuus. Asiakkaan asema terveydenhuollossa. Sosiaali- ja terveysministeriö. Työryhmämuistioita 1998:1. Helsinki: Oy Edita Ab.

Norberg, A. & Athlin, E. (1989) Eating problems in severely demented patients. Issues and ethical dilemmas. Nursing Clinics of North America 24 (3), 781-789.

Norberg, A., Backstrom, A., Athlin, E. & Nordberg, B. (1988) Food refusal amongst nursing home patients as conceptualized by nurse's aids and enrolled nurses: an interview study. Journal of Advanced Nursing 13 (4), 478-483.

Norberg, A. & Hirschfeld, M. (1987) Feeding of severely demented patients in institutions: interviews with caregivers in Israel. Journal of Advanced Nursing 12 (5), 551-557.

Norberg, A., Hirschfeld, M., Davidson, B., Davis, A., Lauri, S., Lin, J.Y., Phillips, L., Pittman, E., Vander Laan, R. & Ziv, L. (1994) Ethical reasoning concerning the feeding of severely demented patients: an international perspective. Nursing Ethics 1 (1), 3-13.

Norberg, A., Norberg, B. & Bexell, G. (1980a) Ethical problems in feeding patients with advanced dementia. British Medical Journal 281, 847-848.

Norberg, A., Norberg, B., Gippert, H. & Bexell, G. (1980b) Ethical conflicts in long-term care of the aged: nutritional problems and the patient-care worker relationship. British Medical Journal 280 (6211), 377-378.

Norup, M., Folker, A., Holtug, N., Jensen, A., Kappel, K. & Nielsen, J. (1998) Decisions about life and death. An empirical study of the position of Danish physicians concering end-of-life decisions. Nordisk Medicin 113 (7), 240-244.

Ogilvie, A. (1980) Sources and levels of noise on the ward at night. Nursing Times 76 (31), 1363-1366.

Oland, L. (1978) The need for territoriality. In H. Yura & M. Walsh (eds.) Human needs and the nursing process. New York: Appleton-Century-Crofts, 97-140.

O'Malley, J.F. (1997) Ultimate patient satisfaction. Designing, implementing or rejuvenating an effective patient satisfaction and TQM program. Healthcare Financial Management Association. New York: McGraw-Hill.

Orem, D. (1991) Nursing: concepts of practice. St Louis: Mosby.

Orenlicher, D. (1992) The illusion of patient choice in end-of-life decisions. Journal of American Medical Association 267, 2101-2104.

Ott, B. (1986) An ethical problem facing nurses: the support of patient autonomy in the do not resuscitate decision. University Microfilms International. Dissertation. Texas Women's University.

Ouslander, J., Tymchuk, A. & Krynski, M. (1993) Decisions about enteral tube feeding among the elderly. Journal of the American Geriatrics Society 41, 70-77.

Owen, A. (1995) Individual practices. Nursing Times 91 (20), 44-46.

Pahlman, I., Hermanson, T., Hannuniemi, A., Koivisto, J., Hannikainen, P. & Ilveskivi, P. (1996) Patient's rights. Three years in force: has the Finnish act on the Status and Rights of Patients materialized? Medicine and Law 15, 591-603.

Palohuhta, A-L. (1995) Omaisen näkemys pitkäaikaissairaan fyysisestä hoitoympäristöstä. Pro gradu-tutkielma, Tampereen yliopisto. Tampere: Hoitotieteen laitos.

Pang, M.C. (1998) Information disclosure: the moral experiences of nurses in China. Nursing Ethics 5 (4), 347-361.

Papanoutsos, E. (1984) Practical philosophy. Athens: Dodoni.

Parrott, K., Burgoon, J.K. & Burgoon, M. & LePoire, B.A. (1989) Privacy between physicians and patients: more than a matter of confidentiality. Social Science and Medicine 29 (12), 1381-1385.

Partanen, M-L. (1993) Laki potilaan asemasta ja oikeuksista. Sosiaalinen Aikakauskirja 2, 5-9.

Patients' Bill of Rights (1973) American Hospital Association. New York.

Pattee, C., Ballantyne, M. & Milne, B. (1997) Epidural analgesia for labour and delivery: informed consent issues. Canadian Journal of Anaesthesia 44 (9), 918-923.

Pearson, A., Hocking, S., Mott, S. & Riggs, A. (1993) Quality care in nursing homes: from the resident's perspective. Journal of Advanced Nursing 18 (1), 20-24.

Peckham, S. (1997) Big ears goes to work. Nursing Times 93 (17), 22-24.

Pellonpää, M. (1996) Euroopan ihmisoikeussopimus. (2. uudistettu painos). Helsingin Lakimiesliiton kustannus. Helsinki: Gummerus.

Phillips, J. (1979) An exploration of perception of body boundary, personal space, and body size in elderly persons. Perceptual and Motor Skills 48 (1), 299-308.

Pinch, W.J.E & Parsons, M.E. (1997) Moral orientation of elderly persons: considering ethical dilemmas in health care. Nursing Ethics 4 (5), 380-393.

Pichler J. (1992) Internationale Entwicklungen in den Patientenrechten. Wien: Böhlau Verlag.

Plati, C. (1997) Geriatric nursing. Athens.

Plank, D.M.P. (1994) Framing treatment options: a method to enhance informed consent. Clinical Nurse Specialist 8 (4), 174-178.

Pluckhan, M. (1968) Space: the silent language. Nursing Forum VII (4), 386-397.

Plumeri, P.A. (1994) Informed consent for upper gastrointestinal endoscopy. Gastrointestinal Endoscopy Clinics of Nort America 4 (3), 455-461.

Politis, C. (1990) Code of medical deontology. Medicine and Law 6, 49-55.

Porter, S (1992) The poverty of professionalisation: a critical analysis of strategies for the occupational advancement of nursing. Journal of Advanced Nursing 7, 720-726.

President's Commission (1982) The President's Commission for the study of ethical problems in medicine and biomedical research: deciding to forego life-sustaining treatment. Washington, DC: US Government Printing Office.

Priami, M. & Plati, C. (1997) Behavioral control of mental patient's. Ethical dimensions. Nosileftiki 3, 272-280.

Proot, I.M., Crebolder, H.F.J.M., Abu-Saad, H.H. & Ter-Meuler, R.H. (1998) Autonomy in the rehabilitation of stroke patients in nursing homes. A concept analysis. Scandinavian Journal of Caring Scieces 12 (3), 139-145.

Proshansky, H., Ittelson, W. & Rivlin, L. (1970) Freedom of choice and behavior in a physical setting. In H. Proshansky, W. Ittelson & L. Rivlin (eds.) Environmental psychology: man and his physical setting. New York: Holt, Rinehart & Winston, 173-183.

Quintana, O. (1993) International bioethics? The role of the Council of Europe. Journal of Medical Ethics 19 (1), 5-6.

Raisch, D. (1993) Barriers to providing cognitive services. American Pharmacy 1993 NS33 (12), 54-58.

Randall, S. (1998) Intimate examinations. The British Journal of Family Planning 24, 83-84.

Raphael, W. (1979) Old people in hospital. London: King Edward's Hospital Fund for London.

Rasmussen, O.V., Henriksen, L.O., Baldur, B. & Hansen, T. (1992) Patientinformation forud for sterilisation. Ugeskr Laeger 154 (14), 2567-2570.

Rawnsley, M. (1980) The concept of privacy. Advances in Nursing Science 2 (2), 25-31.

Re F v West Berkshire Health Authority. (All ER 545). (1989) [On sterilization of women suffering from severe learning disabilities and unable to give consent]

Reizenstein, J. (1982) Hospital design and human behavior: a review of the recent literature. In A. Baum & J. Singer (eds.) Advances in environmental psychology, Vol 4, Environment and health. Hillsdale: Erlbaum, 1085-1087.

Re T (Adult: refusal of treatment) 4 A11 ER 649 (1992)

Richardson, J. & Webber, I. (1998) Ethische Aspekte der Kinderkrankenpflege. Wiesbaden: Ullstein Medical.

Richter, J., Eisermann,M., Bauer, B. & Kreibeck, H. (1998) Entscheidungen und Einstellungen von Krankenschwestern bei der Behandlung chronisch kranker alter Menschen. Pflege (11), 96-99.

Rigatos, G. (1991a) Medical Codes of Ethics. Athens: Epsilon.

Rigatos, G. (1991b) The Hippocratic Oath. Athens: Epsilon.

Riis, P. (1987) Mass screening procedires and programmes. In S. Doxiadis (ed.) Ethical dilemmas in health promotion. Chichester: John Wiley & Sons, 171-182.

Riley, G.J. & Simmonds, R.L. (1992) Informed consent in modern medical practice. Medical Journal of Australia 157 (7), 336-338.

Rittman, M. & Gorman, R. (1992) Computerized databases: privacy issues in the development of the nursing minimum data set. Computers in Nursing 10 (1), 14-18.

Rivera, R., Reed, J.S. & Menius, D. (1992) Evaluating the readability of informed consent forms used in contraceptive clinical trials. International Journal of Gynaecology and Obstetrics 38, 227-230.

Rivero, A. & Galán, T.A. (1998) An international view of patients' rights. Medical ethics and human rights. In Council of Europe. The human rights, ethical and moral dimensions of health care. 120 practical case studies. European Network of Scientific Co-operation on Medicine and Human Rights. Council of Europe Publishing. Germany, 101-109.

Roberto, K., Wacker, R., Jewell, E. & Rickard, M. (1997) Reseident rights. Knowledge of and implementation by nursing staff in long-term care facilities. Journal of Gerontological Nursing 23, 32-40.

Roberts, J. & Gregor, T. (1971) Privacy: a cultural view. In J. Pennock & J. Chapman (eds.) Privacy. New York: The Atherton Press, 199-225.

Roberts, S. (1978) Behavioral concepts and nursing throughout the life span. New Jersey: Prentice-Hall, Englewood Cliffs.

Roberts, S. (1986) Behavioral concepts and the critically ill patient. Norwalk: Appleton-Century-Crofts.

Roosa, W. (1982) Territory and privacy. Residents' views: findings of a survey. Geriatric Nursing 3 (4), 241-243.

Ross C., Frommelt G., Hazelwood L. & Chang R. (1987) The role of expectations in patient satisfaction with medical care. Journal of Health Care Market 7 (4), 16-26.

Routasalo, P. (1997) Touch in the nursing care of elderly patients. Annales Universitatis Turkuensis D 258. University of Turku. Turku: Kirjapaino Pika Oy.

Rowson, R. (1993) Ethics, nurses and patients. London: Scrutari Press.

Royal College of Obstetricians and Gynaecologists (1997) Intimate examinations. Report of Working Party. London: RCOG Press.

Rumbold, G. (1996) Ethics in nursing practice. (2$^{nd}$ ed.). London: Balliere Tindall.

Russell, R., Campbell, A., Allison, G., Caradoc-Davies, T. & Busby, W. (1991) Informed consent for cardiopulmonary resuscitation in elderly patients. New Zealand Medical Journal 1004 (916), 312-313.

Ryhänen, S. & Vaittinen, P. (1994) Vanhuksen kokemus fyysisen hoitoympäristönsä toiminnallisuudesta, yksilöllisyydestä ja sosiaalisuudesta. Pro gradu-tutkielma. Kuopion yliopisto. Kuopio: Yhteiskuntatieteellinen tiedekunta.

Rössler, D. (1996) Editorial: Zur Diskussion über die Bioethik-Konvention. Ethik in der Medizin 8 (4), 167-172.

Saba, V. (1995) Home health care classifications (HHCCs): nursing diagnosis and interventions. In Nursing data systems. ANA. Washington: American Nurses Association, 62-103.

Sainz, A., Quintana, O. & Sánchez, J. (1994) La información médica: el consentimiento informado, fundamentos éticos y legales. Revista de Calidad Asistencial 9 (2), 68-71.

Salmon, P. (1993) Interactions of nurses with elderly patients: relationship to nurses' attitudes and to formal activity periods. Journal of Advanced Nursing 18 (1), 14-19.

Santa-Maria, L. (1982) Perceived intrusions into territorial and personal space as anxiety-producing factors to hospitalized patients: implications to nursing. Phillippines Journal of Nursing II (2), 26-28.

Scanlon, C. & Fleming, C. (1989) Ethical issues in caring for the patient with advanced cancer. Nursing Clinics in North America 24, 977-986.

Schachter, D., Kleinman, I., Prendergast, P., Remington, G. & Schertzer, S. (1994) The effect of psychopathology on the ability of schizophrenic patients to give informed consent. The Journal of Nervous and Mental Disease 182 (6), 360-362.

Scheinin, M. (1992) Johdanto. Teoksessa L. Hannikainen (toim.) Eettiset säännöt. Åbo Akademin ihmisoikeusinstituutti. Turku: Åbo Akademis tryckeri, 2-5.

Schommer, J. & Wiederholt, J. (1995) A field investigation of participant and environment effects on pharmacist-patient communication in community pharmacies. Medical Care 33 (6), 567-584.

Schultz, E. (1977) Privacy: the forgotten need. The Canadian Nurse 73 (7), 33-34.

Schuster, E. (1976a) Privacy and the hospitalization experience. Communicating Nursing Research 7, 153-171.

Schuster, E. (1976b) Privacy, the patient and hospitalization. Social Science and Medicine 10, 245-248.

Schwartz, B. (1968) The social psychology of privacy. The American Journal of Sociology 73, 741-752.

Schwerdt, R. (1998) Eine Ethik für die Altenpflege: ein transdisziplinärer Versuch aus der Auseinandersetzung mit Singer, P., Jonas, H. und Buber, M. Bern: Huber Verlag.

Scott, P.A. (1995) Care, attention and imaginative identification in nursing practice. Journal of Advanced Nursing 21 (1), 196-200.

Scott, P.A. (1997) Imagination in practice. Journal of Medical Ethics 23 (1), 45-50.

Scott, P.A. (1998) Morally autonomous practice? Advances in Nursing Science 21 (2), 69-79.

Seedhouse, D. (1992). The autonomy test: a guide for decision-making. Senior Nurse 12 (2), 37-40.

Segest, E. (1995) The legal position with regard to informed consent in Denmark. Medicine and Law 14 (3-4), 245-254.

Seelye, A. (1982) Hospital ward layout and nurse staffing. Journal of Advanced Nursing 7 (3), 195-201.

Selekman, J. (1989) When the nurse knows and the patient does not: waiting for a diagnosis. Holistic Nursing Practice 4, 1-7.

Shaw, R., Cohen, F., Fishman-Rosen, J., Murphy, M., Stertzer, S., Clark, D. & Myler, R. (1986) Psychologic predictors of psychosocial and medical outcomes in patients undergoing coronary angiolpasty. Psychosomatic Medicine 48, 582-597.

Shotton, L. & Seedhouse, D. (1998) Practical dignity in caring. Nursing Ethics 5, 246-255.

Shotter, J. (1975) Images of man in psychological research. London: Methuen.

Sidaway the Board of Governors of the Bethlem Royal Hospital and the Maudsley Hospital (1984) 1 All England Law Report, 1084, 1018.

Sidenvall, B., Fjellström, C. & Ek, A-C. (1994) The meal situation in geriatric care – intentions and experiences. Journal of Advanced Nursing 20, 613-621.

Siegler, M. (1985) The progression of medicine. From physician paternalism to patient autonomy to bureaucratic parsimony. Archives of Internal Medicine 145 (4), 713 - 715.

Silva, M.C. (1985) Comprehension of information for informed consent by spouses of surgical patients. Research in Nursing and Health 8 (2), 117-124.

Simmel, A. (1950) The sociology of Georg Simmel. New York: Free Press of Glencoe.

Simmel, A. (1971) Privacy is not an isolated freedom. In J. Pennock. & J. Chapman, J. (eds.) Privacy. New York: The Atherton Press, 71-87.

Simón, P. (1995) El Consentimiento Informado y la participación del enfermo en las relaciones sanitarias. Medifam 5, 90-98.

Simón, P. (1996) Bioética y Consentimiento Informado en la Atención Sanitaria. Doctoral tesis. Universidad Santiago de Compostela. Spain. Unpublished.

Simón, P. & Barrio, I. (1995) El consentimiento informado y la enfermería: un modelo integral. Jano 68 (11), 55-64.

Simón, P., Barrio, I. & Concheiro, L. (1996) Legibilidad de los formularios escritos de consentimiento informado. Medicina Clínica 107 (14), 524-529.

Singleton, K.A. & Dever, R. (1991) The challange of autonomy. Respecting the patient's wishes. Dimensions of Critical Care Nursing 10 (3), 160 - 168.

Sklaroff, S. & Atkinson, F. (1987) Disabled patients in acute hospital wards. Clinical Rehabilitation 1, 127-131.

Smith, M. (1996) Data protection, health care and the new European directive. British Medical Journal 312, 197-198.

Snyder, M. (1985) Independent nursing interventions. New York: John Wiley & Sons.

Sommer, R. (1969) Personal space. The behavioral basis of design. Englewood Cliffs: Prentice-Hall.

Sommerseth, E. (1993) Gravides erfaring med informasjonsrutinene ved rutinemessige ultralydundersokelser. Tidsskr Nor Laegeforen 113 (10), 1218-1220.

Sorrell, J.M. (1991) Effects of writing/speaking on comprehension of information for informed consent. Western Journal of Nursing Research 13 (1), 110-122.

Sperl, D. (1996) Qualitätssicherung in der Pflege. 2. Auflage. Hannover: Schlütersche.

Spring, D., Winfield, A., Friedland, G., Shuman, W., & Preger, L. (1988) Written informed consent for IV contrast-enhanced radiography: patients' attitudes and common limitations. AJR 151, 1243-1245.

Spirig, R. (1996) Das ich hierher kommen mußte, haben andere bestimmt. Der Eintritt auf die

Sterbeabteilung. In A. Kesselring (Hg.) Die Lebenswelt der Patienten. Bern: Huber Verlag, 123-153.

Sprung, C.L. & Winick, B.J. (1989) Informed consent in theory and practice: legal and medical perspectives on the informed consent doctrine and a proposed reconceptualization. Critical Care Medicine 17 (12), 1346-1354.

Sriram, T.G., Chatterjee, S., Jain, S., Vergheese , M., Raghavan, K. & Murthy, R. (1989) Opinion survey of physicians on ethical issues in medical research. Journal of the Indian Medical Association 89 (7), 187-190.

Standing Committee of Doctors of the European Community (1987) Principles of the European Medical Deontology. Brussels.

Stanley, B., Guido, J., Stanley, M. & Shortell, D. (1984) The elderly patient and informed consent. Empirical findings. Journal of the American Medical Association 252 (10), 1302-1306.

STM (1986) Sosiaali- ja terveysministeriö. Terveyttä kaikille vuoteen 2000. Suomen terveyspolitiikan pitkän aikavälin tavoite- ja toimintaohjelma. Helsinki: Valtion painatuskeskus.

Stolman, C.J., Castello, F., Yorio, M. & Mautone, S. (1994) Attitudes of pediatricians and pediatric residents toward obtaining permission for autopsy. Archives of Pediatrics and Adolescent Medicine 148, 843-847.

Stratton, J. (1981) Personal space preferences of hospital children for nurse, doctors, family members and strangers. Columbia: University of Missouri.

Streiff, L. (1986) Can clients understand our instructions? Image 18, 48-52.

Strunk, H. (1995) Ethische Regeln der Intensivpflegenden (Ethik-Kodex). Bielefeld: Deutsche Gesellschaft für Fachkrankenpflege e.V.

Störig, H. J. (1987) Kleine Weltgeschichte der Philosophie. Frankfurt: Fischer Taschenbuch Verlag GmbH.

Sugarman, J., McCrory, D. & Hubal, R. (1998) Getting meaningful informed consent from older adults: a structured literature review of empirical research. Journal of American Geriatrics Society 46 (4), 517-524.

Suls, J. & Wan, C. (1989) Effects of sensory and procedural information on coping with stressful medical procedures and pain: a meta-analysis. Journal of Consulting Clinical Psycholoogy 57, 372-379.

Sundstrom, E., Herbert, R. & Brown, D. (1982) Privacy and communication in an open-plan office: a case study. Environment and Behavior 14, 379-392.

Swan, H. & Borshoff, D. (1994) Informed consent: recall of risk information following epidural analgesia in labour. Anaesthesia and Intensive Care 22 (2), 139-141.

Szekely, D.G., Milam, S. & Khademi, J. (1996) Legal issues of the electronic dental record: security and confidentiality. Journal of Dental Education 60 (1), 19-23.

Tadd, W. (Ed.) (1998) Ethical issues in nursing and midwifery practice. Perspectives from Europe. London: MacMillan.

Tajima, T. (1997) Informed consent for patients with advanced cancer. Tokai Journal of Experimental and Clinical Medicine 22 (6), 271-274.

Tanttinen, K. & Rasimus, A. (1994) Terveystietojen tutkimuskäytäntö. Dialogi 1, 32-34.

Taplin, D. (1995) Nursing and informed consent. An empirical study. In G. Hunt (ed.) Ethical issues in nursing. Reprinted. London: Routledge, 21-37.

Tarschys, D. (1998) Preface. In Concil of Europe (1998). The human rights, ethical and moral dimensions of health care. 120 practical case studies. European Network of Scientific Co-operation on Medicine and Human Rights. Councul of Europe Publishing. Germany, 9-10.

Tate, J. (1980) The need for personal space in institutions for the elderly. Journal of Gerontological Nursing 6 (8), 439-449.

Teres, D. (1993) Trends from the United States with end of life decisions in the intensive care unit. Intensive Care Medicine 19 (6), 316-322.

Tervo-Pellikka, R. (1993) Terveydenhuollon potilasasiakirjat. Sosiaalinen Aikakauskirja 2, 15-21.

Tervo-Pellikka, R. (1994) The principles of data protection concerning patient related data in Finland. International Journal of Bio-Medical Computing 35 (Suppl. 1), 39-50.

Thomas, L. & Bond, S. (1996) Measuring patients' satisfaction with nursing: 1990-1994. Journal of Advanced Nursing 23, 747-756.

Thomasma, D.C. (1983) Beyond medical paternalism and patient autonomy: a model of physician conscience for the physician-patient relationship. Annals of Internal Medicine 98 (2), 243-248.

Thomasma, D.C. (1984) Freedom, dependency, and the care of the very old. Journal of The American Geriatrics Society 32 (12), 906-914.

Thompson, J. & Goldin, G. (1975) The hospital: a social and architectural history. New Haven: Yale University Press.

Thompson, I., Melia, K.M. & Boyd, K. (1994) Nursing ethics. (3$^{rd}$ ed.). Churchill Livingstone, Singapore: Longman Singapore Publishers Ltd.

Tingle, J. & Cribb, A. (1995) Nursing law and ethics. Oxford: Blackwell Science.

Tonks, A. (1993) Information management and patient privacy in the NHS. British Medical Journal 307, 1227-1228.

Travers, A., Burns, E., Penn, N., Mitchell, S. & Mulley, G. (1992) A survey of hospital toilet facilities. British Medical Journal 304, 878-879.

Trierweiler, R. (1978) Personal space and itse effects on an elderly individual in a long-term care institution. Journal of Gerontological Nursing 4 (5), 21-23.

Tschudin, V. (1986) Ethics in nursing: the caring relationship. London: Heinemann.

Tymchuk, A. & Ouslander, J. (1990) Optimizing the informed consent process with elderly people. Educational Gerontology 16, 245-257.

Tymchuk, A., Ouslander, J. & Rader, N. (1986) Informing the elderly: a comparison of four methods. Journal of the American Geriatrics Society 34, 818-822.

Ulfig, A. (1997) Lexikon der philosophischen Begriffe. Wiesbaden: Fourier Verlag.

United Kingdom Central Council for Nursing, Midwifery and Health Visiting (1992) Standards for the Administration of Medicines (1992) London: UKKC.

Vaininen, M., Routasalo, P. & Virtanen, T.J. (1999) Rakkaat ja tarpeelliset tavarat. Vanhainkodissa asuvan vanhuksen esineistö. Hoitotieteen laitoksen julkaisuja, Tutkimuksia ja raportteja A:26/1999. Turun yliopisto, Turku: Unipaps.

Varricchio, C. & Jassak, P. (1989) Informed consent: an overview. Seminars in Oncology Nursing 5 (2), 95-98.

Veach, R. (1976) Three theories of informed consent. Philosophical foundations and policy implications. In Belmont Report. Ethical principles and guidelines for the protection of human subjects of research. The National Commission for the Protection of Human Subjects of Biomedical and Behavioral Research. Appendix. Volume II. DHEW Publication No. (OS) 78-0014, 26-1-55.

Veatch, R.M. & Fry, S.T. (1987) Case studies in nursing ethics. Philadelphia: J.B. Lippincott Company.

Vehviläinen-Julkunen, K. Lauri, S. & Kivivirta, L. (1994) Naisten synnytyskokemuksia eri kulttuureissa. Hoitotiede 6 (3), 99-115.

Velecky, L. (1978) The concept of privacy. In J. Younger (ed.) Privacy. Chichester: John Wiley & Sons, 13-34.

Vessey, W. & Siriwardena, A. (1998) Informed consent in patients with acute abdominal pain. British Journal of Surgery 85 (9), 1278-1280.

Viñas, J., Ordoñez, S., Segura, T., Peña, J. & Porta, J. (1999) Valoración del consentimiento informado por parte de los facultativos de un hospital universitario. II Congreso Nacional. Asociación de Bioética Fundamental y Clínica. Madrid.

Volicer, B. & Wynne Bohannon, M. (1975) A hospital stress rating scale. Nursing Research 24 (5), 352-359.

Vollmann, J. (1997) Die Selbstbestimmung von Patientinnen in der sozialpsychiatrischen Praxis. Psychiatrische Praxis 24, 181-184.

Vousden, M. (1987) Private lives. Nursing Times 83 (24), 41-43.

Välimäki, M., Leino-Kilpi, H. & Helenius, H. (1996) Self-determination in clinical practice: the psychiatric patient's point of view. Nursing Ethics 3, 329-344.

Välimäki, M. & Helenius, H. (1996) The psychiatric patient's right to self-determination. A preliminary investigation from the professional nurse's point of view. Journal of Psychiatric and Mental Health Nursing 3 (6), 361-372.

Välimäki, M. (1998) Psychiatric patients' views on the concept of self-determination: findings from a descriptive study. Journal of Clinical Nursing 7, 59-66.

Wade, S. (1995) Partnership in care: a critical review. Nursing Standard, 9 ( 48), 29-32.

Wainwright, P. (1995) The observation of intimate aspects of care. In G. Hunt (ed.) Ethical issues in nursing. London: Routlege, 38-54.

Walker, D.M. (1997) The Scottish legal System: an introduction to the 7th Edition. Study of Scots Law. Edinburgh: W.Green/Sweet & Maxwell.

Warren, S. & Brandeis, L. (1890) The right to privacy. Harward Law Review IV (5), 193-220.

Waters, K. (1994) Getting dressed in the early morning: styles of staff/patient interaction on rehabilitation hospital wards for elderly people. Journal of Advanced Nursing 19, 239-248.

Waterworth, S. & Luker, K.A. (1990) Reluctant collaborators: do patients want to be involved in decisions concerning care? Journal of Advanced Nursing 15 (8), 971-976.

Watkins, M. (1993) Can you tread this emotional high wire? Balancing elderly people's rights against the risks they pose. Professional Nurse 8 (9), 604-608.

Watson, O. (1970) Proxemic behavior: a cross cultural study. The Hague, NL: Monitor & Co.

Watson, R. (1993) Measuring feeding difficulty in patients with dementia: perspectives and problems. Journal of Advanced Nursing 18 (1), 25-31.

Watson, R. (1994) Practical and ethical issues related to the care of elderly people with dementia. Nursing Ethics 1 (3), 151-162.

Watts, D.T., Cassel, C.K. & Hickam, D.H. (1986) Nurses' and physicians' attitudes toward tube-feeding decisions in long-term care. Journal of the American Geriatric Society 34, 607-611.

Weaver, K. (1997) Genetic screening and the right to know. Issues in Law and Medicine 13 (3), 243-281.

Webster's New World Dictionary (1986) New York: Prentice Hall.

Weiss, C.B. (1985). Paternalism modernised. Journal of Medical Ethics 11, 194-197.

Wertz, D. & Fletcher, J. (1998) Ethical and social issues in prenatal sex selection: a survey of geneticists in 37 nations. Social Science and Medicine 46 (2), 255-273.

Westerhall, I. & Phillips, C. (Eds.) (1994) Patients' rights: informed consent, access and equality. Stockholm: Nerenius & Santenus.

Westin, A. (1967) Privacy and freedom. New York: Atheneum.

Westin, A. (1970) Privacy and freedom. New York: Atheneum.

White, M.T. (1998) Decision-making through dialogue: reconfiguring in genetic counseling. Theoretical Medicine Bioethics 19 (1), 5-19.

WHO (1987) Nursing care: summary of a European study. A study of people's needs for nursing care and of the planning, implementation and evaluation of care provided by nurses in two selected groups of people in the European region. Ashworth, Pat. Regional Office for Europe. Copenhagen: World Health Organization.

WHO (1993) Nursing in action. Strengthening nursing and midwifery to support health for all. Sawage, J. (Ed.). WHO, Regional Publications. European series 48. Copenhagen: World Health Organization.

WHO (1994a) Nursing beyond the year 2000. Report of a WHO Study Group. WHO Technical Report Series 842. Geneva: World Health Organization.

WHO (1994b) A declaration on the promotion of patients' rights in Europe. WHO, Regional Office for Europe, Kluwer Law International. The Hague: World Health Organization.

WHO (1996a) European Health Care Reforms. Citizens' Choice and Patients' Rights. WHO, Regional Office for Europe. Copenhagen: World Health Organization.

WHO (1996b) Care in normal birth: a practical guide. Report of technical Working Group. Geneva: World Health Organization.

WHO (1997) European health care reform. Analysis of current strategies. WHO Regional Publications, European series No 72. Copenhagen: World Health Organization.

WHO (1998a) HEALTH21 - An introduction to the health for all policy framework for the WHO European Region. WHO, European Health for All Series No 5. Copenhagen: World Health Organization.

WHO (1998b) HEALTH21 - The health for all policy framework for the WHO European Region. Euripean Health for All Series No 6. Copenhagen: World Health Organization.

Wiens, A. (1993) Patient autonomy in care: a theoretical framework for nursing. Journal of Professional Nursing 9, 95-103.

Willard, C. (1996) The nurses role as patient advocate: obligation or imposition? Journal of Advanced Nursing 24, 60-66.

Willcocks, D., Peace, S. & Kellaher, L. (1987) Private lives in public places. London: Tavistock.

Williams, G.C., Rodin, G.C., Ryan, R.M., Grolnick, W.S. & Deci, E.L. (1998) Autonomous regulation and long-term medication adherence in adult outpatients. Health Psychology 17 (3), 269-276.

Williams, M. (1988) The physical environment and patient care. Annual Review of Nursing Research 6 (3), 61-84.

Wilson, D.M. (1992) Ethical concerns in a long-term tube feeding study. Image: Journal of Nursing Scholarship 24 (3), 195-199.

Wilson-Barnett, J. (1979) Stress in hospital. London: Churchill Livingstone.

Winfield, A., Ford, C., James, A., Heller, R. & Lamballe, A. (1986) Response of patients to informed consent for excretory urography. Urologic Radiology 8, 35-39.

Wolfe, M. (1978) Childhood and privacy. In I. Altman & J. Wohlwill (eds.) Human behavior and environment. Advances in theory and research, Vol 3, Children and the environment. New York: Plenum Press, 175-222.

Wood, M. (1977) Clinical sensory deprivation: a comparative study of patients in single care and two-bed rooms. Journal of Nursing Administration 7, 28-32.

Woods, N. & Falk, S. (1974) Noise stimuli in the acute care area. Nursing Research 23 (2), 144-150.

Wright, R.A. (1987) Human values in health care: the practice of ethics. New York: McGraw-Hill.

Yeo, M. & Dalzier, J. (1991) Autonomy. In M. Yeo (ed.) Concepts and cases in nursing ethics. Peterborough, Ontario: Broadview Press Ltd, 54-85.

Young, J. (ed) (1978a) Privacy. Chichester: John Wiley & Sons.

Young, J. (1978b) Introduction: a look at privacy. In J. Young (ed.) Privacy. Chichester: John Wiley & Sons, 1-10.

Young, A.P. (1994) In the patient's best interest. In G. Hunt (ed.) Ethical issues in nursing. London: Routledge, 164-180.

Younger, K. (1972) Report of the committee on privacy. London: Her Majesty's Stationery Office.

Yura, H. & Walsh, M. (1988) The nursing process. (5th ed.). Norwalk, Connecticut: Appleton & Lange.

Zanecchia, D. (1992) Writing readable informed consent forms. Applied Clinical Trials 1, 52-60.

Ziporyn, T. (1984) Hippocrated meets the data banks: patient privacy in computer age. Journal of the American Medical Association 252 (3), 317-319.

Åkerlund, B.M. & Norberg, A. (1985) An ethical analysis of double bind conflicts as experienced by care workers feeding severely demented patients. International Journal of Nursing Studies 22 (3), 207-216.